Springer

*Berlin
Heidelberg
New York
Barcelona
Budapest
Hong Kong
London
Milan
Paris
Santa Clara
Singapore
Tokyo*

Advances in Critical Care Testing

W. F. List   M. M. Müller   M. J. McQueen   (Eds.)

The 1996 IFCC-AVL Award

With 35 Figures and 109 Tables

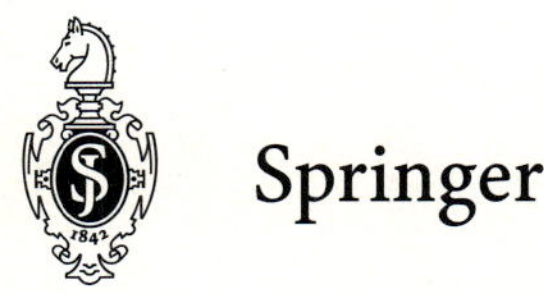

Springer

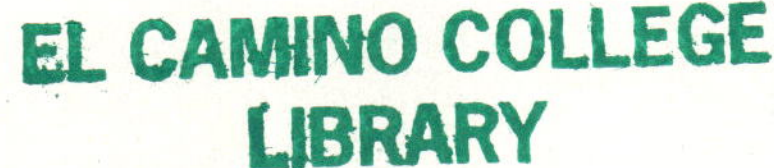

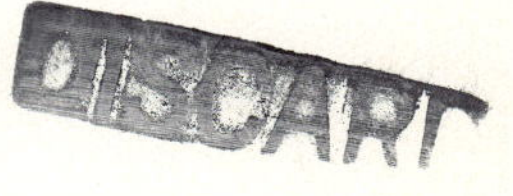

Univ.-Prof. Dr. med. Werner F. List
Universität Graz
Klinik für Anästhesiologie und Intensivmedizin
Auenbruggerplatz 29, A-8036 Graz, Austria

Prof. Dr. med. Mathias M. Müller
Kaiser-Franz-Joseph-Spital
Kundrastraße 3, A-1100 Wien, Austria

Prof. Dr. med. Matthew J. McQueen
McMaster University, Dept. of Laboratory Medicine
732 Barton Street, L8L 2X2 Hamilton, Canada

ISBN 3-540-62590-9 Springer-Verlag Berlin Heidelberg New York

Library of Congress Cataloging-in-Publication Data applied for

Die Deutsche Bibliothek – CIP-Einheitsaufnahme
Advances in critical care testing: the IFCC AVL award 1996; with 109 tables/W. F. List...
(ed.). – Berlin; Heidelberg; New York; Barcelona; Budapest; Hong Kong; London; Milan;
Paris; Santa Clara; Singapore; Tokyo: Springer, 1997
 ISBN 3-540-62590-9 kart.

Production: PRO EDIT GmbH, Heidelberg
Typesetting (Data conversion): K+V Fotosatz GmbH, Beerfelden
Cover Design: design & production GmbH, Heidelberg
SPIN 10560989   19/3133-5 4 3 2 1 0 – Printed on acid-free paper

Preface

This volume on scientific advances in critical care testing compiles a number of clinical and laboratory studies related to critically ill patients that involve new technology, therapy options, application or interpretation of new tests, patient management and cost benefits. There were a total of 340 applicants for this first International Federation of Clinical Chemistry–AVL Award, and from these, National Winners were selected in 26 member countries of the IFCC.

This publication presents the full papers of the ten finalists among the National Winners selected for the international final held in London in July 1996. These ten were chosen by the International Awards Committee of the IFCC. In addition, the editors have decided also to include their choice of the best abstracts from the National Winners, thus giving a broad overview of current research being conducted in the field of critical care medicine among IFCC members.

In keeping with the title of this volume, all major fields of intensive care medicine are represented, including inflammation, infection, stress, hypoxia, ischaemia, cardiology, haemodynamics, blood gases, electrolytes, trace elements, nephrology, gastroenterology and haematology. In addition, there is also a chapter on new technology in critical care testing and on miscellaneous topics.

The paper selected by the IFCC Awards Committee as the best submitted for the 1996 IFCC-AVL Award describes a new test for the biochemical diagnosis of acute aortic damage, which uses an immunoassay to measure smooth muscle-specific myosin heavy chain in plasma. The test has sensitivity and specificity and appears to be a reliable test for the detection of acute aortic disease, aortic dissection and traumatic aortic rupture.

The other finalist papers display a wide spectrum of research interests: leucocyte motion, ventilator-associated pneumonia, glucose-modulated response to endotoxin, neutrophil elastase and C-reactive protein in polytrauma, epidemiological study of activated protein C, expert systems for blood gas interpretation, new technologies for monitoring brain trauma and ischaemia and a simplified left ventricular device for ballon counterpulsation.

The IFCC-AVL Award was sponsored by AVL Medical Instruments, a company whose focus is on critical care testing. The Award was provided in order to promote research and to foster interdisciplinary cooperation in the field of critical care medicine.

The selection of national winners in each country, followed by selection of finalists and eventual winner, involved a considerable amount of work on the part of the individual National Societies and that of the IFCC Awards Committee. Publication of these papers and abstracts required that they be prepared in a standardised format, and this task has been facilitated by Dr. Andrew St John from AVL Medical Instruments, Australia, who acted as an intermediary between authors and the selection committee. The editors would particularly like to express their appreciation to Dr. St John for acting in this capacity and for his meticulous work in helping with the preparation of this publication.

The editors hope that the full papers and selected abstracts provide a good overview of current research interests and of new methods in critical testing.

W.F. List, Graz, Austria

M.M. Müller, Vienna, Austria

M.J. McQueen, Hamilton, Canada

List of Contents

Other Abstracts

Hypoxia – Ischaemia

National Winner

Other Abstracts

Cardiology – Haemodynamics

Finalist

National Winner

Other Abstracts

Blood Gases – Electrolytes – Trace Elements

Finalists

National Winners

Other Abstracts

Nephrology

Other Abstracts

Gastroenterology

National Winners

National Winners

Other Abstracts

List of Paper and Abstract Authors

Dr. L. Ai-lin
Tongji, Department of Anaesthesia,
Tongji Hospital, Tongji Medical
University, Wuhan 430030, PR China

Dr. G.S. Bayer
Department of Plastic and
Reconstructive Surgery, Burns Unit,
University of Vienna Medical School
& Ludwig-Boltzmann Institute
for Experimental Plastic Surgery,
Vienna, Austria

Dr. D.R. Bernard
Laboratorium voor Klinische
Chemie, Universitair Ziekenhuis
Gent, 2B2, De Pintelaan 185,
B 9000 Gent, Belgium

Dr. Lajos Bogar
Department of Anaesthesia
& Intensive Care,
Medical University of Pecs,
PO Box 99, Pecs 7643, Hungary

Dr. B.W. Bottiger
Department of Anaesthesiology,
University of Heidelberg,
Im Neuenheimer Feld 110,
D-69120 Heidelberg, Germany

Dr. Moises Calderon
Passeo de La Soledad 69,
La Herradura, Edo Mex, 53920,
Mexico

Dr. V. Cosic
Department of Biochemistry,
Clinical Centre, Nis, Yugoslavia

Dr. C. de Souza
St Peters Colony, 16 Xavier House,
Manuel Gionsalves Road, Banobia,
Bombay 400050, India

Dr. I. Doyle
Department of Human Physiology,
Flinders University
of South Australia, Bedford Park,
SA 5042, Australia

Dr. Glenn Edwards
Western Diagnostic Pathology,
74 McCoy Street, Myaree,
W Australia 6154, Australia

Dr. A. El Naggar
Faculty of Medicine,
Cairo University Hospital,
Cairo, Egypt

Dr. A. El Sherif
Faculty of Medicine,
Cairo University Hospital,
Cairo, Egypt

Ms. M. Lim Sok Fong
Clinical Biochemistry Laboratories,
Department of Pathology,
Singapore General Hospital,
Outram Road, Singapore

Dr. B. Francois
Service de reanimation polyvalente,
CHU Dupuytren,
2 av Martin Luther King,
87025 Limoges Cedex, France

Dr. G. D. Gomersall
Department Anaesthesia &
Intensive Care, Chinese University
of Hong Kong, Shatin, Hong Kong

Dr. J. Hedstrom
Department of Clinical Chemistry,
University Hospital of Helsinki,
FIN-00290 Helsinki, Finland

Dr. B. Hoppe
University Children's Hospital,
Josef-Stelzmann Str. 9,
D-50931 Cologne, Germany

Dr. S. Ignjatovic
Institute for Medical Biochemistry,
Clinical Centre of Serbia, Polyclinic,
Visegradska 26, 110000 Belgrade,
Yugoslavia

Dr. Timothy Inglis
1 Lower Acreman Street, Sherborne,
Dorset, DT9 3EK, UK

Dr. J. Ishii
Department of Internal Medicine,
Fujita Health University School of
Medicine, Kutsukake-cho, Toyoake,
Aichi 470-11, Japan

Dr. Peter Kirkpatrick
Academic Department of
Neurosurgery, Block A, Level 4,
Addenbrookes Hospital (Box 167),
Hills Road, Cambridge CB2 2QQ,
UK

Dr. A. Kogan
Intensive Care Unit,
Rabin Medical Centre (Beilinson),
Petah Tikva 49100, Israel

Dr. V. Kumar
Department of Paediatrics,
Kalawati Saran Children's Hospital,
LHMC-New Delhi, India

Dr. S. Kunishima
Research Division, Japanese Red
Cross Aichi Blood Centre,
539-3 Minamiyamaguchi, Seto,
Aichi 489, Japan

Mr. B. Lee
Intensive Care Unit,
Royal Melbourne Hospital,
Parkville, Victoria, Australia

Dr. G. Lefevre
Service de Biochimie, Hopital Tenon,
4 Rue de la Chine, F-75970 Paris,
Cedex 20, France

Dr. I. Leonard
Department of Anaesthesia
& Intensive Care,
Mater Misericordiae Hospital,
Dublin 7, Ireland

Dr. Marie-Reine Losser
Department of Anaesthesiology
& Intensive Care,
Lariboisiere University Hospital,
2, Rue Ambroisiere Pare,
75010 Paris, France

Dr. A. W. Lyon
Department of Pathology,
Royal University Hospital,
103 Hospital Drive, Saskatoon, SK,
Canada S7N OW8

Dr. P. Martens
Department of Anaesthesia
and Critical Care, AZ Sint-Jan,
Ruddershove 10, 8000 Brugge,
Belgium

Dr. A. Miller
Department of Neurology,
Carmel Medical Centre,
Haifa, Israel

Dr. P. Myles
Department of Anaesthesia,
Alfred Hospital, Commercial Road,
Prahran, Victoria 3181, Australia

Dr. S. Nangia
B-1/1702, Vasant Kunj,
New Delhi – 110070, India

Dr. C. Pichard
Division of Nutrition, Geneva
University Hospital, 1211 Geneva 14,
Switzerland

Dr. S. Rao
Department of Biochemistry, Sri
Venkateswara Institute of Medical
Sciences, Tirupati, 517507, AP, India

Dr. A. Rizk
Department of Critical Care
Medicine,
Cairo University Hospitals,
Cairo, Egypt

Dr. A. E. Rodriguez
Unidad de investigation, Hospital
General de Elche, Ptda Huertos y
molinos gln, 03202 Elche, Spain

Dr. S. M. Samir
Department of Critical Care
Medicine,
Cairo University Hospitals,
Cairo, Egypt

Dr. T. Samir
Department of Critical Care
Medicine,
Cairo University Hospitals,
Cairo, Egypt

Dr. C. Sandrine
Laboratoire de Biochemie, C.H.U.
Farhat Hached-Sousse 4000, Tunisia

Dr. M. Siggaard-Andersen
Dept. of Genetics,
University of Copenhagen,
Oster Farimagsgade 2A,
DK-1353, Copenhagen, Denmark

Dr. T. Suzuki
3rd Department of Internal
Medicine, Faculty of Medicine,
University of Tokyo, 7-3-1 Hongo,
Bunkyo-ku, Tokyo 113, Japan

Dr. G. Tsongalis
Department of Pathology
& Laboratory Medicine,
Hartford Hospital,
Hartford, CT 06102, USA

Dr. D. Q. Tuan
Intensive Care Unit, Bachmai
Hospital, Hanoi, Vietnam

Dr. P. Vignon
Intensive Care Unit,
CHU Dupuytren, 2 av Martin Luther
King, 87025 Limoges Cedex, France

Dr. D. Weisman
Department of Neonatology, Bnai
Zion Medical Centre, PO Box 4940,
Haifa 31048, Israel

Dr. C. Waydhas
Department of Surgery,
Klinikum Innenstadt, Ludwig-
Maximilians-University of Munich,
Nussbaumstr. 20, 80336 Munich,
Germany

Dr. L. Xuguo
Department of Cardiology,
Yantai Overseas Chinese Hospital,
Yantai 264001, PR China

Dr. R. J. Young
Department of Anaesthesia
& Intensive Care, Prince of Wales
Hospital, Chinese University of Hong
Kong, Shatin, Hong Kong

Dr. P. Zivny
Institute of Clinical Biochemistry
& Diagnostics, Charles University,
Faculty of Medicine, Hradec Kralove,
Czech Republic

Biochemical Diagnosis of Acute Aortic Damage – Diagnosis of Aortic Dissection and Traumatic Aortic Rupture Using an Immunoassay of Smooth Muscle Myosin Heavy Chain

T. Suzuki

Abstract

In the setting of acute medicine, aortic dissection is a very common aortic catastrophe associated with a high mortality and morbidity rate. In the acute trauma setting, aortic rupture is an equally life-threatening event. A reliable biochemical diagnostic method for acute aortic damage would be beneficial to the critical care specialist.

A novel immunoassay of smooth muscle-specific myosin heavy chain was developed. The clinical usefulness for detection of acute aortic diseases, aortic dissection and traumatic aortic rupture was investigated.

Forty patients with aortic dissection were examined. The results showed significant elevations of serum smooth muscle myosin heavy chain during the first 24 h. The sensitivity of the assay was 87% within the first 12 h and 82% within the first 24 h at a cut-off level of 2.5 ng/ml. The specificity of the assay was 97%. Two patients with traumatic aortic rupture also showed significant elevations of serum smooth muscle myosin heavy chain. The immunoassay of serum smooth muscle myosin heavy chain is a rapid and reliable biochemical method in the diagnosis of acute aortic diseases, aortic dissection and traumatic aortic rupture. The potential use of the method in the critical care setting is promising.

Introduction

Vast progress has been made in the last 50 years in cardiovascular biochemical diagnostic testing, beginning with the introduction of the serum transaminase assays in the 1950s [1], followed by assays of enzyme activity in the 1960s, e.g. creatine kinase, lactate dehydrogenase [2, 3], and the clinical applications of assays of structural proteins, e.g. cardiac myosin light chain and troponin [4–8], in the 1970s and 1980s. The role of biochemical testing in clinical cardiovascular medicine has now been firmly established.

In contrast to the expanding availability of cardiac biochemical markers, notably myocardial ones, biochemical assays for vascular diseases have not been available, due in part to a lack of specific markers for vascular diseases. With the recent progress made in the field of vascular biology, molecular markers representative of the vasculature have become available. Characterization of smooth muscle myosin heavy chain, a structural protein found in smooth muscle cells by the authors and by others in the past, has shown that it is specific to the smooth muscle lineage [9–14]. Smooth muscle myosin heavy chain is abundantly expressed in the aortic wall, and detection of the smooth muscle-specific component released into the circulation from the damaged aortic wall by the immunoassay [15] has proven to be useful in the diagnosis of aortic diseases, aortic dissection and traumatic aortic rupture [16–18].

Immunoassay of Serum Smooth Muscle Myosin Heavy Chain

A double monoclonal sandwich enzyme immunoassay was developed to measure serum smooth muscle myosin heavy chain. The details of the immunoassay have been described elsewhere [17].

Methodology

BALB/c mice were immunized with human uterus myosin emulsified in complete Freund's adjuvant at 2-week intervals. Following six immunizations and an additional booster injection, splenocytes obtained from the mouse with the highest titer as assessed by enzyme-linked immunosorbent assay (ELISA) [19] were fused with mouse myeloma cells by standard methods [20]. The supernatant of the cultured hybridoma was screened for anti-smooth muscle myosin antibody production by ELISA, and the specific antibody-producing hybridoma cells were cloned by limiting dilution.

Monoclonal antibodies were produced in ascitic fluid of BALB/c mice, primed with pristane and purified. The combination of paired antibodies with the highest assay sensitivity was used for the double monoclonal antibody sandwich assay. Measurements were completed within 4 h.

Technical Properties

The assay showed reliable detection of smooth muscle myosin heavy chain in human serum. The sensitivity of the assay was approximately 0.4 ng/ml, with a measuring range up to approximately 50 ng/ml. Cross-reactivity with cardiac, skeletal or platelet myosin was negligible at less than 0.1%.

Analysis of 75 healthy individuals showed smooth muscle myosin heavy chain levels in normal human sera to be 0.9±0.1 ng/ml.

Statistical Analysis

All results are presented as mean±SE. Unless noted otherwise, comparison between means of two independent samples was performed by the two-tailed unpaired t test, and analysis of multiple groups was performed with analysis of variance (ANOVA), adjusted by the Bonferroni/Dunn method. Statistical significance was defined as $p<0.05$.

Clinical Applications

To determine the clinical usefulness of the immunoassay, clinical studies have been conducted. With hopes that the immunoassay could detect diseases of the aorta, pilot studies were conducted which have indeed shown the immunoassay to be clinically useful in the diagnosis of aortic dissection and aortic rupture [16–18].

Diagnosis of Aortic Dissection

Aortic dissection is a very common aortic catastrophe [21]. In the United States, it is estimated that there are approximately 2000 new cases of aortic dissection reported each year [22–25]. If left untreated or undetected, there is a mortality rate of 21% within the first 24 h alone [25]. In the acute setting, diagnosis of aortic dissection is not always readily feasible. Often, the patient may not tolerate extensive diagnostic examination. The presenting signs and symptoms may also be obscure, especially in patients with haemodynamic deterioration, a common complication of the disease. Detecting the aortic catastrophe from among the range of events concurrently occurring in the acute critical care setting may often prove to be a difficult task. Even in the presence of the newer diagnostic modalities, e.g. magnetic resonance imaging, transoesophageal echocardiography, which have greatly contributed to the increased accuracy of ante-mortem diagnosis of the disease [26, 27], the diagnosis may remain undetected. Unfortunately, aortic dissection is still frequently missed today [28]. By detecting the smooth muscle-specific component released into the circulation from the damaged aortic wall with the immunoassay, the presented results have shown the immunoassay of smooth muscle myosin heavy chain to be useful in the diagnosis of aortic dissection.

Serum smooth muscle myosin heavy chain levels were examined prospectively in 40 patients with aortic dissection, and the characteristics of the assay were determined.

Table 1 summarizes the demographic and clinical characteristics of the enrolled patients with aortic dissection.

The baseline patient characteristics showed patients with non-significant age and sex differences. The initial serum smooth muscle myosin heavy chain levels did not show any statistical relationship with any of the clinical parameters, e.g. age, sex, diagnosis. The time course of serum smooth muscle myosin heavy chain levels in the 40 patients with aortic dissection is shown in Fig. 1. Analysis of smooth muscle myosin heavy chain levels with other biochemical parameters did not show significant correlation with smooth muscle myosin heavy chain, e.g. leucocyte count, haematocrit, erythrocyte sedimentation rate, the

Table 1. Patient characteristics for aortic dissection

Patients (n)	
Total	40
Male	28
Female	12
Mean age (years)	
Total	66.3±1.5
Male	65.7±1.9
Female	67.6±2.5
Mean admission time (h)[a]	9.0±1.6
Diagnosis: aortic dissection (n)	
DeBakey type I	16
DeBakey type II	6
DeBakey type III (A,B)	14

[a] Time after onset.

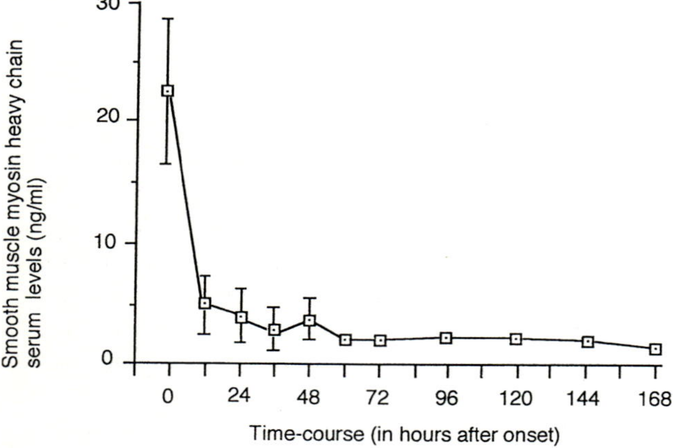

Fig. 1. Time course of serum smooth muscle myosin heavy chain levels in patients with aortic dissection (n=40). Note that peak levels are at onset. A rapid reduction in levels is seen during the first 24 h

acute phase reactant C-reactive protein, aspartate transaminase, alanine transaminase, lactate dehydrogenase, total bilirubin, blood urea nitrogen, creatinine levels and creatine kinase or MB fraction.

At a cut-off value of 2.5 ng/ml, the assay showed a sensitivity of 87% during the first 12 h after onset, which was reduced to 82% at 24 h. The sensitivity during the first 24-hour period should allow for detection in patients receiving medical attention during this time period. The specificity of the assay – as the ability to differentiate patients from healthy subjects – was 97%.

Analysis of the lesion site according to DeBakey classification in relation to serum smooth muscle myosin heavy chain levels showed significant reductions in smooth muscle myosin heavy chain levels within the first 12 h for DeBakey type II as compared to other lesions (DeBakey type I, 6.9±2.3 ng/ml, $n=7$; type II, 38.6±19.6 ng/ml, $n=4$; type III, 6.1±2.9 ng/ml, $n=9$; $p<0.05$). Analysis at 72 h showed similar characteristics. DeBakey type II lesions are localized to the proximal aortic root, in contrast to types I and III, which involve widespread damage beginning at the proximal and distal aortic roots, respectively; the characteristic reductions in such localized lesions may be suggestive of a semi-quantitative role of the assay.

A semi-quantitative role was suggested by the remarkable reductions in localized lesions, although localization of the lesion did not prove possible from one-point initial measurements alone; thus serial measurements may prove useful in the assessment of the pathogenic state, e.g. localization, resolution.

Additionally, the levels were not augmented in patients with renal failure, a common complication associated with aortic dissection. This characteristic of serum smooth muscle myosin heavy chain levels should allow for reliable measurements in patients with renal dysfunction; augmentation of levels by renal function is a problem often encountered in biochemical testing, e.g. creatine kinase.

Diagnosis of Aortic Rupture

Aortic rupture is most often associated with a traumatic aetiology and is found in association with patients who have had a motor vehicle accident [29, 30]. Avulsion of arterial branches from sites of fixation is considered to be the pathogenic mechanism of the insult, with the site of injury very often being localized to the vicinity of the aortic isthmus. Due to the nature of the disease, high morbidity and mortality rates are associated with the aortic damage [31], and associated complications are commonly found [32]. As patients with blunt trauma in the acute setting often present with a multitude of signs and symptoms, and as they are often unstable, the diagnosis may indeed be difficult to ascertain. Despite its low sensitivity and specificity, widening of the mediastinum on chest X-ray is still considered to be one of the characteristic findings suggestive of the disease. The pathogenesis of the disease is considered to originate at the adventitia with lacerations or transections of the outer aortic wall as the site of origin further leading to medial disruption. As the disease is rare, only a limited number of patients have been examined.

Two patients with aortic rupture were examined. The demographic and clinical characteristics of the enrolled patients are shown in Table 2. Both showed elevations at 13.4±10.3 ng/ml, and both had traumatic aetiology caused by motor vehicle collisions with multiple associated traumatic injuries; both were haemodynamically stable, and aortic rupture was suspected by widening of the mediastinum on chest X-ray following admission. The diagnosis was confirmed by ultrasonography, computed tomography and aortography in both cases; subsequent surgical intervention was also performed.

Table 2. Patient characteristics for aortic rupture

Patient	Sex	Age (years)	Aetiology	Associated complications
Patient no. 1	Male	54	Trauma, motor vehicle accident	Multiple fractures of the lower extremities, traumatic subarachnoid haemorrhage
Patient no. 2	Female	50	Trauma, motor vehicle accident	Multiple fractures of the nose, five ribs, forearm and pelvis, haemothorax, retroperitoneal haematoma

As shown in Fig. 2, the serum levels showed a characteristic time profile similar to that of aortic dissection.

As the assay is specific to smooth muscle myosin heavy chain, levels are not elevated in patients with damage to other muscles, e.g. heart, skeletal muscle, which is a disadvantage in the trauma setting, in which there is often concurrent skeletal damage and occasionally myocardial damage.

At present, in patients with a history of a high-risk background, e.g. rapid deceleration in vehicle collisions, or with signs suggesting traumatic aortic rupture, e.g. marked widening of the mediastinum on chest X-ray, the assay could be of benefit as an adjuvant method to aid in the clinical judgment and management of the disease. Early detection by immediate testing may be beneficial in the clinical management of similar cases.

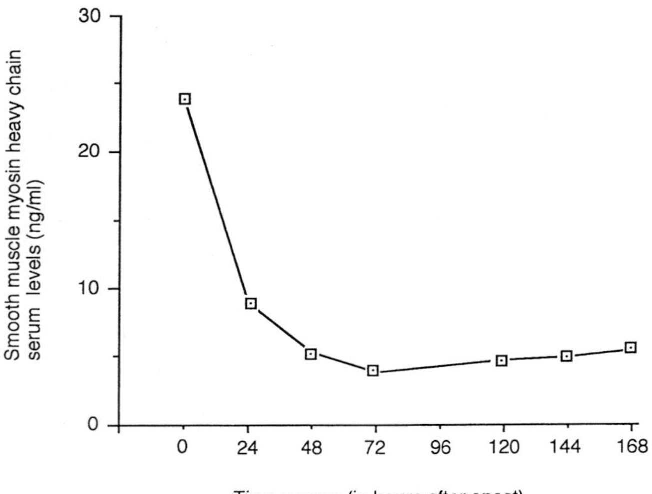

Fig. 2. Serial measurements of serum smooth muscle myosin heavy chain levels in a representative patient with aortic rupture. Note that peak levels are at onset

Conclusion

Diagnosis of aortic catastrophes has remained a challenge for critical care-oriented physicians and surgeons. As the signs and symptoms of aortic damage are often obscure, mimicking signs and symptoms of other confusing diseases or remaining undisclosed among the vast range of events simultaneously occurring in the critical care setting, aortic diseases are sometimes overlooked or diagnosed too late. Despite recent advances in clinical management, e.g. newer imaging diagnostic techniques and the introduction of surgical treatment, early diagnosis and initiation of treatment have remained the key factors in improved survival. To further improve upon the clinical approaches and management of acute aortic diseases, a simple, fast and accurate method for screening of aortic damage would indeed be beneficial. Immunoassay of smooth muscle myosin heavy chain has proven to be a useful tool for diagnosis of aortic dissection and aortic rupture in the critical care setting.

The assay shows tremendous clinical possibilities, providing an easy, fast and accurate method for screening of aortic dissection and aortic rupture. In the critical care setting, as one parameter of the clinical assessment, the method may play an adjuvant role in the diagnosis along with other available diagnostic methods. At institutions which do not have diagnostic instruments available or in cases in which extensive testing is not readily feasible, the biochemical method may provide a highly useful tool for screening aortic dissection or aortic rupture.

References

1. LaDue JS, Wroblewski F, Karmen A (1954) Serum glutamic oxaloacetic transaminase activity in human acute transmural myocardial infarction. Science 120:497–499
2. Sorensen NS (1963) Creatine phosphokinase in the diagnosis of myocardial infarction. Acta Med Scand 174:725–734
3. Kibe O, Nilsson NJ (1967) Observations on the diagnostic and prognostic value of some enzyme tests in myocardial infarction. Acta Med Scand 182:597–610
4. Katoh H, Sugi M, Chino S et al (1992) Development of an immunoradiometric assay kit for ventricular myosin light chain I with monoclonal antibodies. Clin Chem 38:170–171
5. Trahern CA, Gere JB, Kurauth GH, Bigham DA (1978) Clinical assessment of serum myosin light chains in the diagnosis of acute myocardial infarction. Am J Cardiol 41:641–645
6. Cummins B, Auckland ML, Cummins P (1987) Cardiac-specific troponin-I radioimmunoassay in the diagnosis of acute myocardial infarction. Am Heart J 113:133–144
7. Katus HA, Remppis A, Looser S, Hallermeier K, Scheffold T, Kubler W (1989) Enzyme linked immunoassay of cardiac troponin T for the detection of acute myocardial infarction in patients. J Mol Cell Cardiol 21:1349–1353
8. Nagai R, Ueda S, Yazaki Y (1979) Radioimmunoassay of cardiac myosin light chain II in the serum following experimental myocardial infarction. Biochem Biophys Res Commun 86:683–688
9. Nagai R, Larson DM, Periasamy M (1988) Characterization of a mammalian smooth muscle myosin heavy chain cDNA clone and its expression in various smooth muscle types. Proc Natl Acad Sci USA 85:1047–1051

10. Nagai R, Kuro-o M, Babij P, Periasamy M (1989) Identification of two types of smooth muscle myosin heavy chain isoforms by cDNA cloning and immunoblot analysis. J Biol Chem 264:9734–9737

11. Kuro-o M, Nagai R, Tsuchimochi H et al (1989) Developmentally regulated expression of vascular smooth muscle myosin heavy chain isoforms. J Biol Chem 264:18272–18275

12. Aikawa M, Silvam PN, Kuro-o M et al. (1993) Human smooth muscle myosin heavy chain isoforms as molecular markers for vascular development and atherosclerosis. Circ Res 73:1000–1012

13. Yanagisawa M, Hamada Y, Katsuragawa Y, Imamura M, Mikawa T, Masaki T (1987) Complete primary structure of vertebrate smooth muscle myosin heavy chain deduced from its complementary DNA sequence. J Mol Biol 198:143–157

14. Miano JM, Cserjesi P, Ligon KL, Periasamy M, Olson EN (1994) Smooth muscle myosin heavy chain exclusively marks the smooth muscle lineage during mouse embryogenesis. Circ Res 75:803–812

15. Katoh H, Suzuki T, Hiroi Y et al (1995) Diagnosis of aortic dissection by immunoassay for circulating smooth muscle myosin. Lancet 345:191–192

16. Suzuki T, Katoh H, Watanabe M et al (1996) A novel biochemical method for aortic dissection – the results of a prospective study using an immunoassay of smooth muscle myosin heavy chain. Circulation 93:1244–1249

17. Katoh H, Suzuki T, Yokomori K et al. (1995) A novel immunoassay of smooth muscle myosin heavy chain in serum. J Immunol Methods 185:57–63

18. Suzuki T, Maekawa K, Morita H et al. Biochemical diagnosis of traumatic aortic rupture – using a serum assay of smooth muscle myosin heavy chain (submitted)

19. Sugi M, Kato H, Fujimoto M et al (1987) Monoclonal antibodies to human beta interferon: characterization and application. Hybridoma 6:313–320

20. Kohler G, Milstein C (1975) Continuous culture of fused cells secreting antibody of predefined specificity. Nature 256:495–497

21. Miller DC (1985) Acute dissection of the aorta: continuing need for earlier diagnosis and treatment. Mod Con Cardiovasc Dis 54:51–55

22. Anagnostopoulos CE, Prabhakar MJS, Kittle CF (1972) Aortic dissections and dissecting aneurysms. Am J Cardiol 30:263–273

23. Wheat MW Jr (1980) Acute dissecting aneurysms of the aorta: diagnosis and treatment – 1979. Am Heart J 99:373–387

24. Roberts WC (1981) Aortic dissection: anatomy, consequences, and causes. Am Heart J 101:195–214

25. Hirst AE, Johns VJ Jr, Kime SW Jr (1958) Dissecting aneurysms of the aorta: a review of 505 cases. Medicine 37:217–279

26. Cooke JP, Safford RE (1986) Progress in the diagnosis and management of aortic dissection. Mayo Clin Proc 61:147–153

27. Nienaber CA, von Kodolitsch Y, Nicolas V et al (1993) The diagnosis of thoracic aortic dissection by noninvasive imaging procedures. N Engl J Med 328:1–9

28. Spittell PC, Spittell JA Jr, Joyce JW et al (1993) Clinical features and differential diagnosis of aortic dissection: experience with 236 cases (1980 through 1990). Mayo Clin Proc 68:642–651

29. Turney SZ, Rodriguez A (1990) Injuries to the great thoracic vessels. In: Turney SZ, Rodriguez A, Cowley RA (eds) Management of cardiothoracic trauma. Williams and Wilkins, Baltimore, pp 229–260

30. Ben MY (1993) Rupture of the thoracic aorta by broadside impacts in road traffic and other collisions: further angiographic observations and preliminary autopsy findings. J Trauma 35:363–367

31. Smith RS, Chang FC (1986) Traumatic rupture of the aorta: still a lethal injury. Am J Surg 152:660–663

32. Ochsner MJ, Hoffman AP, DiPasquale D et al (1989) Pelvic fracture as an indicator of increased risk of thoracic aortic rupture. J Trauma 29:1376–1379

Inflammation – Infection – Stress

Leucocyte Motion During Gravity Sedimentation of Whole Blood

L. Bogár, J.A. Horváth, and M. Tekeres

Abstract

The rate of leucocyte accumulation was measured in the upper half of the Westergren tube after 1 h of gravity sedimentation of whole blood. The increment of leucocyte concentration, i.e. leucocyte antisedimentation rate (LAR), was determined as a percentage of the original leucocyte count. LAR was measured in 15 patients after surgical intervention in the early postoperative period. C-reactive protein (CRP), the erythrocyte sedimentation rate (ESR) and the severity score of systemic inflammatory response syndrome (SIRS) were also assessed simultaneously. There was a significant positive correlation between SIRS scores and LAR (r, 0.493; $p<0.01$). However, the correlation between SIRS scores and ESR and between SIRS scores and CRP was not significant (r, 0.346, NS; and r, 0.017, NS, respectively). In conclusion, LAR is superior to ESR and CRP in monitoring systemic inflammation (septic complications) in patients after thoracic and abdominal tumour resection.

Introduction

Erythrocyte sedimentation rate is widely accepted as a non-specific test to assess the effect of some acute-phase proteins on erythrocyte aggregation [1]. The factors that determine blood sedimentation have been thoroughly investigated; however, little is known about the behaviour of leucocytes during erythrocyte aggregation and sedimentation.

Previously, we modified the Westergren erythrocyte sedimentation technique for measuring LAR [2]. Briefly, the sodium citrate-anticoagulated whole blood samples were filled into vertically positioned silicone tubes; after 1 h of sedimentation, the concentration of leucocytes was determined in the upper half of the tube. LAR was calculated as the increment of leucocyte concentration in the upper half of the sedimentation tube. Assuming that the leucocytes are distributed evenly in the blood column prior to the start of sedimentation, LAR indicated the percentage of leucocytes and leucocyte subpopulations which had crossed the middle line of blood column. The normal range of LAR is between 0% and 20%.

In our previous study, we found a significant negative correlation between leucocyte adhesiveness and LAR and a significant positive correlation between ESR and LAR [2]. In vitro pre-treatment of blood samples with water-soluble prednisolone or lidocaine resulted in a significant, concentration-dependent diminishment of LAR [2]. In an other study, we demonstrated that LAR was superior to ESR in predicting progress of disease in out-patients suffering from chronic lymphocytic leukaemia or myeloma [3]. In the present study, our aim was to investigate LAR in the patients who were at risk of developing postoperative systemic inflammatory (septic) complications in a surgical intensive care unit.

Patients and Methods

The mean age of 15 patients was 63 ± 14 years (SD); nine were male, and six were female. Oesophageal tumour resection was performed in seven patients, and eight underwent total or subtotal gastric resection due to neoplastic disease. All were treated in a surgical intensive care unit, and two out of 15 patients died, one on the 12th and the other on the 21st postoperative day. Informed consent was obtained from each of them preoperatively. Blood samples were aspirated through central venous lines into silicone-coated 6.25 ml glass tubes containing 1.25 ml sodium citrate (concentration, 105 mol/l; Becton Dickinson Vacutainer, Systems Europe, Meylan, France). ESR, LAR and CPR measurements (quantitative immunoturbidimetry, antiserum; Orion Diagnostics, Helsinki, Finland) and capillary blood gas analysis (AVL 995; AVL List GmbH, Biomedical Instruments, Graz, Austria) were performed on the first, third and fifth or sixth postoperative days.

Leucocyte Antisedimentation Study

Westergren blood sedimentation technique was modified for measuring leucocyte motion during gravity sedimentation of whole blood [2]. The vertically positioned silicone tubes with parameters identical to those of the original technique (internal diameter, 2.5 mm; height of blood column, 200 mm) were filled with 0.98 ml sodium citrate-anticoagulated whole blood (Figs. 1, 2). After 1 h of sedimentation, ESR was recorded and the upper half of the blood column was aspirated via a plastic tube 0.5 mm in diameter attached to the sedimentation tube at the level of 100 mm. The increment of leucocyte count in the post-sedimentation sample was measured with an automatic cell counter (Coulter Counter CBC5, Coulter Electronics Ltd., Luton, United Kingdom) and expressed as a percentage, taking the pre-sedimentation leucocyte concentration as 100%. The percentage of leucocytes which had crossed the middle line of the sedimentation tube was measured as follows:

$$LAR = (A/B - 1) \times 100$$

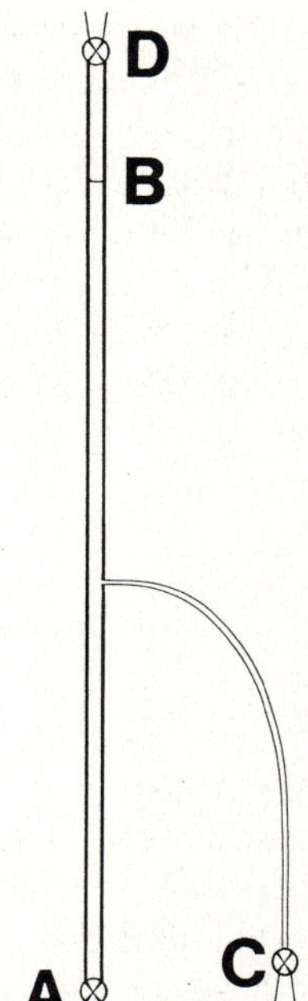

Fig. 1. Westergren sedimentation tube modified for measurement of leucocyte antisedimentation rate. *A*, tap for filling up the sedimentation tube; *B*, upper surface of blood column at 200 mm; *C*, tap connected to the drain-tube attached to the sedimentation tube at 100 mm; *D*, tap for cleaning the sedimentation tube by aspiration

where A is the leucocyte concentration in the upper half of the blood column after 60 min of gravity sedimentation, and B is the pre-sedimentation leucocyte concentration.

Sedimentation measurements were carried out at room temperature ($22\pm1^{\circ}C$), and preparations were started within 30 min after blood sampling.

Assessment of Inflammatory Complications

SIRS scores (0–4) were determined retrospectively according to the American College of Chest Physicians and the Society of Critical Care Medicine Consensus Conference [4] in all patients, using the worst recordings on the first, third and fifth or sixth postoperative days (one point for each criterion):
- Temperature $>38^{\circ}C$ or $<36^{\circ}C$
- Heart rate >90 beats/min
- $PaCO_2$ <32 mmHg
- Peripheral leucocyte count >12|000 cells/mm^3 or <4000 cells/mm^3

A Student's *t* test was used for statistical evaluations, and $p<0.05$ was considered significant.

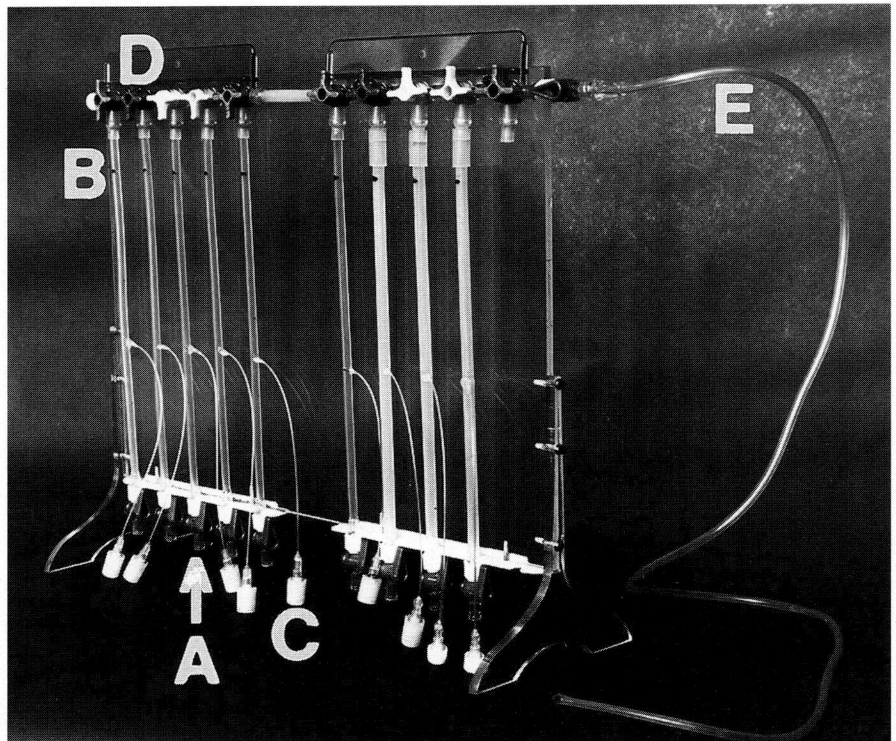

Fig. 2. Device used for measuring leucocyte antisedimentation rate. *A*, taps for filling up the sedimentation tubes; *B*, upper surface of blood columns at 200 mm; *C*, taps connected to the drain-tubes attached to the sedimentation tube at 100 mm; *D*, taps for cleaning the sedimentation tube by aspiration; *E*, tube attached to a suction system

Results

There was no consistent change in the measured parameters as a function of postoperative time. However, LAR was in positive correlation to SIRS scores (r, 0.493; $p<0.01$), and LAR increased significantly at SIRS scores 3 and 4 compared to score zero ($p<0.05$ and $p<0.01$, respectively; Fig. 3A). The equation derived from the data shown on Fig. 3A is as follows:

$$\text{SIRS score} = (0.05 \times \text{LAR}) - 0.77$$

There was no significant correlation between SIRS scores and ESR (r, 0.346, NS; Fig. 3B) and between SIRS scores and CRP concentration (r, 0.017, NS; Fig. 3C).

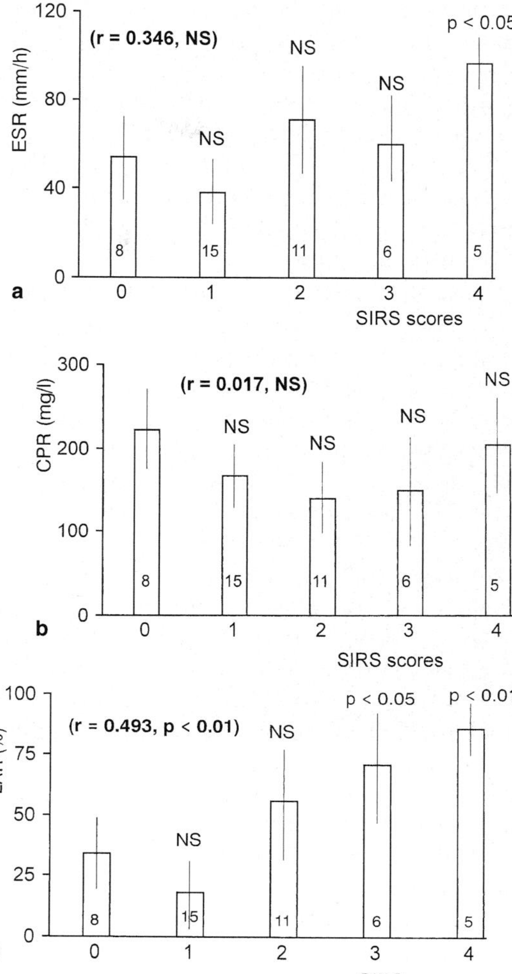

Fig. 3a–c. All data were grouped into five categories according to the severity scores of systemic inflammatory response syndrome (*SIRS*). Changes in **a** erythrocyte sedimentation rate (ESR), **b** C-reactive protein (CRP) and **c** leucocyte anti-sedimentation rate (LAR) are shown with the SIRS scores (mean ± SD). Significance was in relation to SIRS score 0; *r*, correlation coefficient; the number of measurements is shown on the *bars*

Discussion

Whole blood sedimentation is a three-phase process. In the first phase, the erythrocytes form aggregates (rouleau and sphere formation), and in the second phase, the spheres of uniform size settle according to the Einstein-Stokes equation while the cells and plasma are separating. In the third phase, the cells sediment into a dense column [5]. Leucocytes are pushed by the aggregating erythrocytes towards the vertical tube wall, where they ascend and finally settle on the interface between erythrocytes and plasma. Several factors can alter the ascension of leucocytes in a vertical tube (velocity of erythrocyte sedimentation, plasma viscosity, plasma density and leucocyte characteristics, i.e. cell size, shape, specific gravity, tendency to form aggregates).

Furthermore, the change in the differential white blood cell count can alter the mean cell density (mature granulocytes have a higher specific gravity than band forms). The issue of leucocyte flotation and/or ascension raises some questions related to the reliability of leucocyte isolation procedures by gravity sedimentation: Are we sampling the same leucocyte population if we isolate leucocytes from different blood samples even for intraindividual comparison? Perhaps the leucocytes of interest remain in the red cell column despite dextrane-facilitated sedimentation? These questions have to be answered in the future.

SIRS originates from the presence of infectious foci or non-infectious tissue damage. Whatever the primary pathogenic process, SIRS involves activation of monocytes and polymorphonuclear leucocytes by primary inflammatory mediators (bacterial endotoxins, tumour necrosis factor, interleukins) and by secondary mediators (complement fragments, platelet-aggregating factor) [6]. In an in vitro experiment, it has been demonstrated that the density of activated leucocytes (eosinophils) is less than that of non-activated cells [7]. This observation can explain our recent results, assuming that the process of SIRS enhances leucocyte activation and thus decreases cell density, which results in an increased LAR. In another human, double-blind, placebo-controlled, crossover experiment, Evans et al. [8] demonstrated increased leucocyte density after patients with mild stable asthma had been pre-treated with inhalational corticosteroid. We published similar results from a previous study: LAR decreased in a dose-dependent manner after in vitro pre-treatment with water-soluble prednisolone [2].

Preparative procedures and storage of leucocytes can cause cell activation and swelling [9]. Avoiding isolation methods and using whole blood samples may improve quality control of leucocyte functional tests, particularly for clinical studies. Although LAR is measured in whole blood and is highly dependent on ESR and other non-leucocytic factors (erythrocyte count, plasma density and viscosity), our recent study proved that LAR is more sensitive to systemic inflammation than ESR. Further controlled trials are required to establish the value of LAR (sensitivity and specificity) in early prediction of SIRS and infectious complications in critically ill patients.

Conclusions

This is the first study ever to prove that the leucocyte antisedimentation test provides new information on the characteristics of circulating leucocytes in critically ill patients. This publication describes the method for measuring leucocyte antisedimentation as a new quality of leucocytes.

Circulating leucocytes promptly react to different exogenous and endogenous inflammatory challenges. Thus leucocyte activation can be the earliest sign of an acute-phase reaction. Considering this fact, it is plausible that the change in the functional state of circulating leucocytes can be the earliest warning sign of systemic or secondary organ complication in severely traumatized (i.e. surgical) and/or infected patients treated in intensive care units. This study demonstrated that LAR significantly correlates with SIRS in patients after thoracic and/or abdominal tumour resection.

The leucocyte antisedimentation test does not require any cell isolation procedures, and it is therefore highly probable that the unwanted activation of leucocytes is avoided. However, the activation process during 1 h of sedimentation can only be due to the effect of inflammatory mediators already present in the patient's own blood sample.

Finally, the LAR test is easy to perform, reproducible, inexpensive and less time-consuming than any other leucocyte functional test.

Acknowledgement. This study was supported by the Soros Foundation. Authors are indebted to Mrs. L. Szepes, Ms. G. Dombai and the late Mr. K. Spitl for their excellent technical assistance.

References

1. International Council for Standardization in Haematology (Expert Panel on Blood Rheology) (1993) ICSH recommendations for measurement of erythrocyte sedimentation rate. J Clin Pathol 46:198–203
2. Bogár L (1993) Leucocyte antisedimentation rate: a novel method for evaluation of leucocyte activation. Clin Hemorheol 13:291 (abstr)
3. Bogár L, Sárosi I, Nagy Á (1995) Leucocyte antisedimentation in acute myocardial infarction and in hematological malignancies. Biorheology 32:117–118 (abstr)
4. American College of Chest Physicians/Society of Critical Care Medicine Consensus Conference (1992) Definitions for sepsis and organ failure and guidelines for the use of innovative therapies in sepsis. Crit Care Med 20:864–874
5. Fabry TL (1987) Mechanism of erythrocyte aggregation and sedimentation. Blood 70:1572–1576
6. Lamy M, Deby-Dupount G (1995) Is sepsis a mediator-inhibitor mismatch? Intensive Care Med 21:S250-S257
7. Zoratti EM, Sedgwick JB, Bates ME et al (1992) Platelet-activating factor primes human eosinophil generation of superoxide. Am J Respir Cell Mol Biol 6:100–106
8. Evans PM, O'Connor BJ, Fuller RW et al (1993) Effect of inhaled corticosteroids on peripheral blood eosinophil counts and density profiles in asthma. J Allergy Clin Immunol 91:643–650
9. Nash GB, Jones JG, Mikita J et al (1988) Effects of preparative procedures and of cell activation on flow of white cells through micropore filters. Br J Haematol 70:171–176

Is Ventilator-Associated Pneumonia the Result of Exposure to Host-Derived Inflammatory Mediators?

T.J.J. Inglis, G.S.H. Lee, and M. Kowolik

Abstract

Pneumonia is the major infectious cause of mortality and morbidity in the mechanically ventilated, critically ill patient, yet the condition remains difficult to treat successfully and currently available preventive strategies are, at best, only moderately effective.

We have proposed that ventilator-associated pneumonia (VAP) results from the dissemination of tracheal tube biofilm into the lungs by ventilator gas flow [1]. More recently, we recognised the prevalence of effete neutrophils in the biofilm [2] and documented potent formyl-methionyl-leucyl-phenylalanine (FMLP)-stimulated chemiluminescence following biofilm exposure [3].

We have now examined luminal biofilms and their washings for free myeloperoxidase, which we found in almost all specimens examined. The presence of myeloperoxidase in tracheal tube biofilm, on used suction catheters and in the respiratory circuit supports our hypothesis that the biofilm is formed by progressive accretion of respiratory secretions during suction catheterisation and that it acts as a source of host-derived inflammatory material for eventual dissemination into the lungs.

Our results provide us with a new set of laboratory end points with which to investigate the epidemiology of VAP and subsequently assess the impact of novel preventive strategies we have designed.

Introduction

Despite decades of research, pneumonia continues to make a substantial contribution to the mortality and morbidity of critically ill patients. Nosocomial pneumonia; known in the mechanically ventilated intensive care patient as VAP, is difficult both to accurately diagnose and to successfully treat. Interest has therefore turned in recent years to preventive strategies such as selective decontamination. However, no preventive intervention attempted has been more than partially successful. Improvements are only likely to be on the basis of a better understanding of the pathogenesis of the disease, particularly the earlier stages that are more susceptible to novel interventions.

Following the observation that bacteria in tracheal tube biofilm could be disseminated many centimetres from the tip of the tracheal tube by ventilator gasflow, we proposed that dissemination of tracheal tube biofilm during mechanical ventilation might be a means of bacterial colonisation of the lungs in critically ill patients [1]. Simulation studies on the particles generated by fluid dynamic events within the tracheal tube during conventional mechanical ventilation then showed that their size and momentum were suitable for dissemination deep within the lower respiratory tract [4]. A further study on the distribution of biofilm on the luminal surfaces of tracheal tubes used in critically ill patients showed features suggestive of fluid dynamic phenomena within the tube and pointed to a possible role for the suction catheter in formation of the biofilm [5].

Although the above studies provided some circumstantial evidence for the role of flow phenomena in the colonisation stage of the pathogenesis of VAP, our attention was focused on processes involving bacteria, particularly gram-negative bacilli originating in the patient's gastrointestinal tract [6–8]. Only when the effect of tracheal tube biofilm was tested for FMLP-stimulated chemiluminescence and found to be a potent promoter was the presence of host-derived inflammatory mediators actively considered [3]. In a recent study using confocal laser microscopy to examine undisturbed tracheal tube biofilm, we have found neutrophils in varying stages of decay throughout the luminal biofilm and present in almost all tubes studied [2].

In view of the above considerations, we assayed myeloperoxidase in luminal biofilm from a consecutive series of tracheal tubes used in patients in our surgical intensive care unit and found the neutrophil enzyme present in easily measurable concentrations in the majority of specimens [9]. Having found myeloperoxidase present in tracheal tube biofilms, and knowing that ventilator gasflow might deliver the enzyme into the lower respiratory tract along with the bacteria we had been studying, we set out to investigate how widely myeloperoxidase could be found within the parts of the respiratory circuit adjacent to the tracheal tube.

In the present study, we aimed to determine the following: (a) how widely neutrophil contents were spread within the proximal circuit, (b) whether there was any evidence to support deposition of the biofilm by tracheal suction catheter passage, and (c) whether there was anything to suggest dissemination of neutrophil contents simultaneous to gram-negative bacteria in vivo.

Materials and Methods

Specimens were obtained from consecutive patients admitted to a surgical intensive care unit for prolonged mechanical ventilation (longer than 24 h expected at time of admission). The lowermost 2 cm of the first tracheal suction catheter used each day was cut into a sterile 20-ml container. Before the ventilator tubing angle piece was replaced after tracheal suction, a sterile dry cotton swab was carefully inserted and used to swab the inside surface of the removable cap. Both samples were collected every morning that the patient remained connected to the ventilator. After disconnection for weaning (or death), the tracheal tube would be removed and kept for laboratory analysis. All specimens were placed in a refrigerator ($0°-4°C$) immediately after collection and transported to the laboratory for processing shortly afterwards.

Sample Preparation

The suction catheter tip lumen was cut into two 1 cm sections, the lumina of which were sealed with melted wax to avoid contamination by their contents. The lowermost 1 cm segment was used for bacteriological culture, and the upper segment was used for myeloperoxidase assay.

The cotton swab was cut into 2.0 ml sterile saline and its contents resuspended by vortexing at minimum speed for 10 s.

The external surface of the tracheal tube was cleaned with cotton wool soaked in ethanol; 2.0 ml sterile water was then allowed to run under gravity over the full length of the tube's lumen from connector to tip and collected into a sterile container. Following this, two 1 cm lengths of tube were cut with a sterile scalpel below the inflatable cuff and at the top of the tube, respectively. At both levels, the biofilm was sampled with a sterile cotton swab, which was run gently round the entire luminal circumference and then used to inoculate a 5% sheep blood agar plate (Becton Dickinson, Heidelberg, Australia). The remaining biofilm was scraped from the luminal surface with a sterile wooden spatula and resuspended in 2.0 ml sterile water, as above.

Myeloperoxidase Assay

Myeloperoxidase was assayed using a colorimetric technique [10]. In this assay, the substrate was 0.003% hydrogen peroxide, and the indicator was saturated O-dianisidine HCl (Sigma Chemical Company, St Louis, Missouri, USA). A standard curve was obtained by serial dilution of a suspension of freshly obtained normal human neutrophils (Fig. 1), and results were read as absorbance at 460 nm on a spectrophotometer (model 601, Shimadzu, Japan) against a reagent-containing blank.

Bacterial Culture

The suction catheter tip was inoculated by gently rolling it over the surface of the agar plate. All other specimens were inoculated onto agar plates by sterile cotton swab.

Bacteria were identified to species level using standard phenotypic methods after 18 h of incubation at $37°C$ on fresh sheep blood agar, as described above.

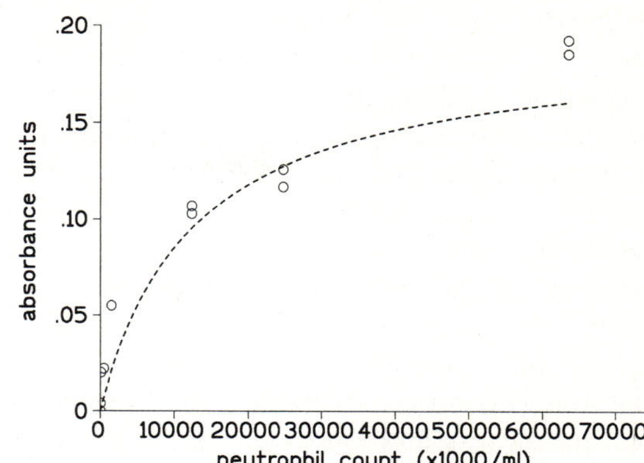

Fig. 1. Myeloperoxidase colorimetric assay standard curve, showing 95% confidence intervals

Genotypic Typing

Genotypic comparison was made by a polymerase chain reaction (PCR)-based typing method using a primer pair for repetitive extragenic palindromic sequences (REPS), known to be present in the majority of gram-negative bacilli. This method was used in a previous epidemiological study in intensive care patients [7]. Briefly, four to five colonies of the strain to be typed were suspended in 50 µl sterile distilled water and boiled for 5 min; 1.2 µl boiled cells were then added to 10.8 µl reagent mixture (primer pair for REPS; REP1R-I 5' III-ICg-ICG-ICA-TCI-ggC-3', REP2R 5' ICg-ICT-TAT-CIg-gCC-TAC 3', Bio-Synthesis Inc., Lewisville, USA; dNTP at a final concentration of 200 µM each; Taq polymerase 2u, Promega, USA; dimethylsulphoxide at a final concentration of 10%, Merck, USA; Triton-X-100 at final concentration of 1%, Sigma, St. Louis, USA; bovine serum albumin, 2.50 mg/ml, Idaho Technology Inc., USA; 10×PCR reaction buffer containing 500 mM Tris-HCl, Sigma, and 20 mM MgCl$_2$, Merck, at a pH of 8.3), mixed and sealed into glass capillary tubes. Thermal cycling was performed with an air thermal cycler (Idaho Technologies, USA): initial denaturation at 95°C for 3 min, then 30 cycles (denaturation at 90°C for 0 min, annealing at 45 C for 1 min, elongation at 65°C for 8 min), and final elongation at 65°C for 16 min. Capillary tubes were scored and their contents transferred to Eppendorf tubes; 3 µl buffer was added. A 13 µl aliquot was used to fill a well in a 1% agarose gel and run for 30 min at 80 V, 2 h at 20 V and finally 1 h at 80 V. The gel was stained with ethidium bromide for 20 min and destained in water for the same period.

Statistical Analysis

Statistical calculations were performed using C-stat (version 1.0, 1991, Cherwell Scientific, Oxford, UK) running under DOS 5.0 (Microsoft Corp., USA). Tests performed included descriptive statistics, Mann-Whitney U test and calculation of Spearman's rank correlation coefficient.

Results

Detectable levels of myeloperoxidase were found in all ten patients' proximal respiratory circuits. Absorbance readings were well in excess of the lower 95% confidence limit on the lowest standard used in the majority of suction catheters and angle piece specimens (Table 1). Although the assay was only semiquantitative, there was a high degree of correlation between absorbance readings in specimens from both sites taken on the same day (Spearman R, 0.8003, T, 8.4425, df, 40, $p<0.001$). Positive myeloperoxidase assays were obtained from both sites in the majority of patients within 24 h of admission to the intensive care unit (Table 2) and antedated the appearance of gram-negative bacilli at either site in seven patients. The remaining three patients had positive results for myeloperoxidase and culture at these sites simultaneously. No patients had positive results for gram-negative bacilli before the suction catheter or angle piece became myeloperoidase positive.

Myeloperoxidase was also detected in luminal biofilms from both upper and lower portions of tracheal tube and in the washings from the same tubes (Table 3). In two cases, the readings obtained from specimens of washings were very high and were similar to the highest readings obtained from the biofilm at the lower end of the tube (Fig. 2). There was, however, no significant correlation between absorbance readings at any of these sites or with readings from suction catheter and angle piece specimens obtained immediately before removal of the tracheal tube.

Table 1. Absorbance readings for myeloperoxidase colorimetric assay, showing negative control, suction catheter and angle piece results (absorbance units)

	Specimens (n)	Absorbance (absorbance units)	
		Range	Mean
Negative control	2	0.00–0.004	0.002
Suction catheter	42	0.0160–0.220	0.1194
Angle piece	42	0.0040–0.205	0.1102

Table 2. Duration of intensive care stay before positive results were obtained in suction catheter and angle piece for both myeloperoxidase and gram-negative bacilli

Specimen	Positive result	Patients (n)	Duration of stay (days)	
			Range	Mean
Suction catheter	Myeloperoxidase	10	1	1
	Gram-negative bacilli	7	1–7	3
Angle piece	Myeloperoxidase	10	1	1
	Gram-negative bacilli	5	1–6	3

Table 3. Myeloperoxidase assay results (absorbance) in specimens from tracheal tubes used in ten consecutive intensive care patients

Specimen	Patients (n)	Absorbance (absorbance units)	
		Range	Mean
Washings	10	0.083–1.20	0.285
Lower tube	10	0.112–1.25	0.349
Upper tube	10	0.047–0.148	0.107

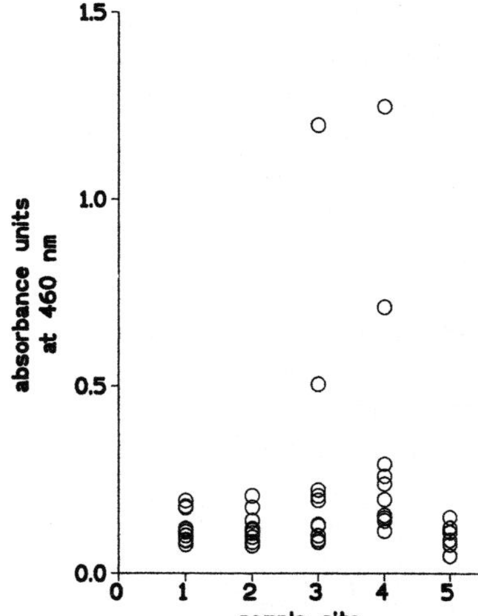

Fig. 2. Myeloperoxidase assay results in tracheal tube specimens and related suction catheter and angle piece specimens. Sample sites: *1*, suction catheter tip; *2*, ventilator circuit angle piece; *3*, washing from luminal tracheal tube biofilm; *4*, lower tracheal tube biofilm specimen; *5*, upper tracheal tube biofilm specimen

Gram-negative bacilli were isolated from two or more different sites in the same patient in six of the ten consecutive patients investigated (Table 4). PCR-based typing confirmed that there was at least one set of identical isolates in all six patients, and in some cases more than one type strain was present. In three of the six patients, where bacteria were present in washings, identical bacteria were present in the biofilm from the same tracheal tube, and the same three patients also had identical bacteria isolated from the suction catheter tip. In two cases, identical bacteria were found in the angle piece and subsequently in washings from the used tracheal tube. These two patients also had the same isolates present in tracheal tube biofilm and suction catheter specimens. Two patients had identical isolates present at all sites but washing and at all sites but the angle piece, respectively.

Table 4. Sites from which identical gram-negative bacilli were isolated, as confirmed by polymerase chain reaction (PCR)-based repetitive extragenic palindromic sequences (REPS) typing

Isolate	Site				
	1	2	3	4	5
Klebsiella pneumoniae	* ————	* ————	* ——— *		
Pseudomonas aeruginosa	* ————	* ——/	/——— *		
Klebsiella pneumoniae	* ——–/	/—— *	——— *		
Pseudomonas aeruginosa	* —— —–/		/——— *		
Pseudomonas aeruginosa	* ————	* ————	* ——— *	———— *	
Klebsiella oxytoca	*——–/	/——— *	——— *	———— *	

1, suction catheter tip; 2, angle piece; 3, tracheal tube washings; 4, lower tracheal tube biofilm; 5, upper tracheal tube biofilm.

Discussion

The mechanically ventilated patient is subjected to an abrupt inrush of oxygen approximately 12–16 times per minute. The tracheal tube is the point in the entire respiratory circuit with the narrowest cross-sectional area and is therefore subject to the greatest pressure changes during the ventilator cycle. Even in a straight, narrow-bore tube lined with a viscoelastic fluid (such as respiratory secretions or tracheal tube biofilm), gasflow would be expected to induce a slower flow in the lining fluid. At higher gas velocity or when the lining layer is either less viscous or thicker, there is a greater probability of disruption to the gas–liquid interface, with consequent fragmentation, and production of an aerosol. In a respiratory circuit with sudden directional changes (the angle piece and curvature of tracheal tube), intermittent flow, variable thickness luminal lining layer (tracheal tube biofilm) and sudden alterations in cross-sectional area (tracheal tube tip into trachea), turbulent flow is all the more likely to cause aerosolisation of the luminal biofilm.

It is not possible to analyse the contents of airborne particulate matter discharged from the tip of the tracheal tube during use in a critically ill patient. We therefore have to extrapolate from what can be obtained during the expiratory phase of ventilation. It has already been shown that particulate matter and viable bacteria similar to those present in tracheal tube biofilm can be found on the patient side of ventilator filters placed at the Y-piece of a ventilator circuit [1]. Consideration of the fluid dynamics of the ventilator circuit suggests that the angle piece, being the point at which the first abrupt change of gasflow direction occurs during expiration, should be a suitable point for sampling fragments of tracheal tube biofilm aerosolised during expiration. However, in patients capable of coughing, there remains the possibility that respiratory secretions from lower down the respiratory tract might be deposited in a similar manner on the inside of the angle piece.

The principle aim of this study was to investigate the extent of biofilm distribution within the proximal respiratory circuit of mechanically ventilated intensive care patients. The finding of positive myeloperoxidase assays on specimens from suction catheter tips and ventilator angle pieces within the first few days after admission to the intensive care unit supports an early dissemination within the circuit.

The presence of myeloperoxidase inside the angle piece, whose 90° bend ensures inertial impaction of exhaled particulate matter during the expiratory phase of ventilation, is consistent with airborne dissemination of fragmented biofilm. The inside of the angle piece does not come into direct contact with the suction catheter, but it is possible in some cases that respiratory secretions adherent to the outer surface of the suction catheter tip might contaminate the seating of the angle piece, and therefore the outer portion of the area swabbed, when the angle piece is replaced. Every effort was made to avoid this kind of contamination in the present study, but a much larger study is required to ensure that this apparent relationship is sustained.

Our analysis of myeloperoxidase on suction catheters and, after their removal, the patients' tracheal tube is consistent with observations we have made previously implicating the process of suction catheterisation in the formation of tracheal tube biofilm. However, as before, this is no more than circumstantial evidence. More compelling evidence is the identical bacterial isolates from biofilm and suction catheter in all six patients with gram-negative bacilli isolated at more than one site. Either these isolates were deposited on the luminal surface of the tracheal tube by the respective suction catheter tip, or the suction catheter was contaminated by bacteria already present on the tube and probably deposited by prior suction catheterisation. Although outside the scope of the present study, previous work of ours [7] suggests that these bacteria originate in the patient's endogenous enteric flora and track down the outer surface of the tracheal tube. The subsequent action of passing a suction catheter back and forth in respiratory secretions containing inter alia neutrophils and bacteria would thus charge the lower end of the tracheal tube as if it were a muzzle-loading musket, ready for the next ventilator-induced blast of in-rushing oxygen.

It is apparent from these observations and previous studies [2, 9] that, although often present together, neutrophil contents, such as myeloperoxidase, and gram-negative bacilli are not necessarily co-existent in tracheal tube biofilm. Moreover, it appears that dissemination of myeloperoxidase antedates dissemination of bacteria within the proximal respiratory circuit. Myeloperoxidase is the only neutrophil product to be studied so far, but other toxic neutrophil products such as elastase, cationic proteins and free radicals clearly require detailed study in this setting. Repetitive exposure of the pulmonary epithelial surface to such a potent mixture of inflammatory stimulants may explain the natural history of VAP, without recourse to bacterial invasion.

There is debate over the role of a variety of specific inflammatory mediators in the pathogenesis of acute inflammatory lung injury in the critically ill patient, particularly acute respiratory distress syndrome and multiple organ system failure. However, elastases are thought to contribute to some forms of lung injury [11], and instillation of chemotactic peptides has long been known to promote an inflammatory reaction in the lung [12]. Furthermore, exposure to superoxide dismutase promotes pulmonary inflammation [13], and oxygen metabolites have been shown to damage the lungs of laboratory animals [14]. It is possible that the addition of gram-negative bacilli to this mixture, and particularly their lipopolysaccharides, might augment the toxic effect of these host-derived inflammatory mediators.

In the above preliminary investigation, we have found neutrophil products and gram-negative bacilli disseminated widely in the proximal respiratory circuit of mechanically ventilated intensive care patients within days of admission. We have found evidence to support the formation of tracheal tube biofilm by deposition of respiratory secretions during suction catheterisation. If confirmed in a larger clinical study, these observations may lead to a better understanding of the pathogenesis and thus the prevention of VAP.

Acknowledgements. We would like to thank all our colleagues who have helped us reach this point in our investigations. We are particularly grateful to Mike Sherratt and Mike Patton (both formerly of University of Leeds, UK) for assistance with the neutrophil chemiluminescence that opened up this line of study, and to John Candlish for suggesting an inexpensive method for the myeloperoxidase assay. We also thank our nursing colleagues in the Surgical Intensive Care Unit at the National University Hospital, Singapore, for willingly collecting all the specimens we requested. This work was supported in part by research project grants from the National University of Singapore.

References

1. Inglis TJJ, Millar MR, Jones JG, Robinson DA (1989) Tracheal tube biofilm as a source of bacterial colonization of the lung. J Clin Microbiol 27:2014–2018
2. Inglis TJJ, Lim TM, Tang C, Ng ML, Hui KP (1995) Structural features of tracheal tube biofilm formed during prolonged mechanical ventilation. Chest 108:1049–1052
3. Inglis TJJ (1995) New insights into the pathogenesis of ventilator-associated pneumonia. J Hosp Infect 30 [Suppl]:409–413
4. Inglis TJJ, Jones JG, Paxton S (1993) Penetration of an aerosol, produced by film atomization, through the carinal bifurcation. Br J Anaesth 70:527–531
5. Inglis TJJ (1993) Evidence for dynamic phenomena in residual tracheal tube biofilm. Br J Anaesth 70:22–24
6. Inglis TJJ, Sproat LJ, Sherratt MJ, Hawkey PM, Gibson JS, Shah MV (1992) Gastroduodenal dysfunction as a cause of gastric bacterial overgrowth in patients receiving mechanical ventilation of the lungs. Br J Anaesth 68:499–502
7. Inglis TJJ, Sherratt MJ, Sproat LJ, Gibson JS, Hawkey PM (1993) Gastroduodenal dysfunction and bacterial colonisation of the ventilated lung. Lancet 341:911–913
8. Inglis TJJ, Sproat LJ, Sherratt MJ, Hawkey PM, Gibson JS (1993) Staphylococcal pneumonia in ventilated patients: a twelve month review of cases in a UK intensive care unit. J Hosp Infect 23:207–210
9. Choong YL (1995) Structural features and contents of tracheal tube biofilm. BSc (Hons) dissertation, Department of Microbiology, National University of Singapore

10. Bradley PB, Christensen RD, Rothstein G (1982) Cellular and extracellular myeloperoxidase in pyogenic inflammation. Blood 60:618–622
11. Janoff A (1985) Elastases and emphysema: current assessment of the protease-antiprotease hypothesis. Am Rev Respir Dis 132:417–433
12. Kreutzer DL, Desai U, Orr W, Showell H, Ward PA (1979) Induction of acute inflammatory reactions in lung following intrapulmonary instillation of preformed chemotactic peptides and purified complement components. Chest 755:2595–2625
13. McCormick JR, Harkin MM, Johnson KJ, Ward PA (1981) The effect of superoxide dismutase on pulmonary and dermal inflammation. Am J Pathol 102:55–61
14. Johnson KJ, Fantone JC, Kaplan J, Ward PA (1981) In vivo damage of rat lungs by oxygen metabolites. J Clin Invest 67:983–992

Glucose Metabolism Modifies Experimental Endotoxin Shock

M.-R. Losser and D. Payen

Abstract

Glucose metabolism dysregulation is frequent during sepsis. However, glucose regulates cytokine production in human monocytes. Glucose is the major energy substrate for various cells, including vascular and immunocompetent cells. In addition, nitric oxide (NO) plays an important role in haemodynamic pattern and inflammation during sepsis, and its biosynthesis may interact with glucose metabolism. One can therefore expect that glucose availability may interfere with the response to endotoxin (EDTX) challenge in vivo. We compared the haemodynamic and metabolic response, i.e. arterial glucose, lactate and blood gases, and the inflammatory response, i.e. tumour necrosis factor (TNF)-α release, NO_2/NO_3 production, in normally fed rabbits, in rabbits after a 24-h fast, and in acutely glucose-loaded, fasting rabbits.

A 24-h fast depleted the glycogen stores in liver (measured by ethanol precipitation) compared to fed animals, whereas 4 g glucose infused via the portal vein in these fasting animals increased the glycogen stores within 30 min. After EDTX, fed animals experienced a hypokinetic shock. Lactic acidosis occurred together with hyperglycaemia and elevated $PaCO_2$, indicating an increased rate of glycolysis. In contrast, EDTX in fasting animals elicited a hyperkinetic shock without metabolic alterations. Glucose load before EDTX in fasting animals restored a shock pattern similar to fed conditions. When we compared arterial glucose kinetics in septic and control animals, there was no difference in glucose disappearance, whereas lactate production, initially driven by glucose supply, was increased together with $PaCO_2$ after EDTX. This suggests that there is no specific EDTX-induced impairment in glucose uptake at this early stage of sepsis, but a specific stimulation of glycolysis. Arterial TNF-α (cytotoxicity on LM clone of murine fibroblasts) showed classical kinetics with a peak 1 h after EDTX. This response was fourfold amplified by glucose loading compared to the two other groups. NO production assessed by plasma NO_2/NO_3 (Griess reaction) only increased in fed animals. In fasting rabbits, EDTX did not increase circulating nitrates in the presence or absence of glucose supply.

Glucose availablity is an important determinant of septic shock pattern. There was no simple correlation between TNF-α and NO_2/NO_3 release and haemodynamics.

Introduction

Hyperglycaemia is a common feature of severe sepsis in humans [2], but the impact of hyperglycaemia on cardiovascular patterns and immune response has not yet been evaluated. Elevated plasma glucose concentration has been demonstrated to modify vascular reactivity, suggesting a direct effect of glucose on endothelial functions and smooth muscle physiology [12, 25, 26]. Glucose is also the major energy substrate for immunocompetent cells, such as monocytes and macrophages. Glucose uptake has been shown to be tremendously increased in activated immunocompetent tissues and macrophages, especially in the liver [17]. Glucose can regulate IL-1β production by human endotoxin-stimulated monocytes in culture, mainly via energy supply [19]. Hyperglycaemia during sepsis results mainly from enhanced hepatic glucose production [28] and peripheral insulin resistance [24], leading the liver to be considered as a key organ in such situations [20]. The liver is also an immunocompetent organ, since it contains the greatest proportion of resident macrophages and is also a source of cytokines [7] and NO [4] in acute inflammation.

Based on this, one can expect that modifications of the glucose balance will have an impact on metabolism, cytokine levels, NO release and systemic and liver haemodynamics. This hypothesis has been tested in a previously described EDTX shock in anaesthetized, non-resuscitated rabbits [21] under different glucose conditions. The results suggest a predominantly metabolic control of the cardiovascular modifications usually observed during EDTX-induced inflammation.

Materials and Methods

New Zealand White rabbits (Charles River, France) weighing 2.2±0.2 kg (mean±SD) were studied in accordance with approved guidelines for the care and use of laboratory animals. The EDTX shock model has been previously described [21]. Briefly, 1200 µg of a mixture of three types of EDTX (*Escherichia coli*, *Salmonella enteritidis* and *Salmonella minnesota*, 400 µg each; Sigma Chemical Co., St. Louis, MO) were injected over 1 min through a marginal ear vein at the end of the surgical preparation.

Animal Preparation

Anaesthesia was induced by intravenous pentobarbital sodium (30 mg/kg) and maintained by a continuous infusion (10 mg/h). The animals were also paralysed (pancuronium bromide, 0.2 mg/kg per h), underwent tracheostomy and were ventilated with 100% oxygen (Rodent Ventilator 638, Harvard Apparatus, Boston, MA). Apyrogen 0.9% saline solution with 0.2 mEq/ml bicarbonate was continuously infused (4 ml/kg per h) throughout the experiment.

A 16-gauge catheter was inserted into the right carotid artery and connected to a pressure transducer (Abbott, North Chicago, IL) linked to a pressure monitor (CGR, Thomson Telco, France). A 20-MHz pulsed Doppler flow velocity probe with an inside diameter (ID) of 5.0 or 6.0 mm was positioned on the ascending aorta, through a superior sternotomy. After a midline laparotomy, 20-MHz probes were placed around the proper hepatic artery (ID, 1.3 mm) and around the portal vein beneath its bifurcation (ID, 4.0 mm). The probes were connected to a multichannel directionally pulsed Doppler flowmeter (Engineering Department of Baylor College of Medecine, Houston, TX) [13]. Mean arterial pressure (P_{Am}) and aortic, hepatic arterial and portal venous blood flow velocities (V_{Ao}, V_{HA} and V_{PV}, in cm/s) were continuously measured and recorded every 15 min on a paper graph monitor (Gould ES 1000).

Study Design

Animals had free water access, and modification of glucose availability was obtained by the following protocol:
- Fed group ($n = 16$): normally fed animals with standard pellets (47.5% carbohydrates, 12% cellulose, 4% fat, 19% proteins)
- Fasting group ($n = 11$): animals fasting for 24 h before initiation of experimental procedures
- Glucose-loaded, fasting animals ($n = 11$) and controls ($n = 5$): the fasting animals had a 24-gauge catheter inserted in an ileal vein through which 8 ml of a 50% dextrose apyrogen solution was injected over 30 min at the end of surgery (corresponding to 2 g glucose/kg).

All groups except the control group one received EDTX. After a recovery period of 30 min following surgery, three consecutive haemodynamic measurements over 30 min were performed to assess the stability of the preparation. The observation period lasted for 180 min following EDTX or saline injection.

Hepatic Glycogen Content

To ensure that the protocol conditions had markedly influenced glucose metabolism, the hepatic glycogen content was measured in separate animals without EDTX injection. The liver tissue samples (1.5–2.0 g) were freezed-clamped using liquid nitrogen and stored at $-30°C$ for subsequent glycogen content measurement; after protein solubilization using 40% KOH ($100°C$, 30 min) and an overnight precipitation at $4°C$ by ethanol, the glycogen pellet was dissolved in 2N HCl and hydrolyzed to glucose ($100°C$, 3 h). The glucose content was then determined enzymatically [16]. The glycogen content was expressed as the equivalent glucose per g wet liver tissue weight (glucose/g wet).

Metabolic Measurements

Plasma glucose and lactate levels (0.5 ml arterial blood samples collected in sodium fluoride/potassium oxalate-containing tubes) were measured using a spectrophotometric technique (Ektachem C-700 Analyzer, Johnson and Johnson, Strasbourg, France). Arterial samples (0.3 ml heparinized blood) were collected at 30-min intervals for blood gas analysis (Radiometer ABL-30, Copenhagen, Denmark).

Tumour Necrosis Factor Assay

In selected animals, blood samples were collected on pyrogen-free ethylene diamine tetra-acetate (EDTA)-containing glass tubes, centrifuged at 5°C and stored at –40°C. Plasma TNF-α activity was measured by a specific in vitro cell cytotoxicity assay [3] using actinomycin D-treated murine fibroblast LM cells (American Type Culture Collection, Rockville, MD). Cytotoxicity was detected using a tetrazolium dye technique. The plates were read at 570 nm on microtitre plate reader (model 650, Dynatech Laboratories, Alexandria, VA) against n-propyl alcohol blanks. A standard curve relating cell cytotoxicity to doses of recombinant human TNF-α was used to quantify TNF-α activity in the samples.

Nitrite/Nitrate Asssay

NO release was assessed by deterimining plasma levels of the NO derivatives NO_2 and NO_3 (NOx, µmol/l). Arterial NOx plasma concentrations were determined using an automated analyser according to Green et al. [11] with minor modifications [30]. The absorbance was spectrophotometrically measured at 546 nm.

Statistical Analysis

Results were expressed as mean±SE. Differences at t_0 between the different groups were tested by unpaired t test. In the animals with glucose supply, paired t tests were used to compare the acute modifications induced by glucose infusion. Comparisons over time between the groups after EDTX or saline were performed by analysis of variance (ANOVA) for repeated measures and one grouping factor. When the analysis was significant, comparisons of the mean values were tested by Sheffe's test. Intragroup differences were tested by one-way ANOVA for repeated measures. Differences with $p<0.05$ were considered significant.

Results

Impact of the Nutritional Regimen on Baseline Values

Liver glycogen stores were depleted in animals after a 24-h fast compared to those on normal feeding (Table 1, $p<0.01$); pH, bicarbonate and lactate levels were also lower (see Fig. 2, $p<0.05$), but glycaemia and haemodynamic variables were similar (Table 2). Thirty minutes after the end of glucose infusion in fasting animals, the hepatic glycogen content increased ($p<0.05$, Table 1) with hyperglycaemia ($p<0.01$, Table 3), lactate and $PaCO_2$ increases ($p<0.05$, Table 3) leading to a pH decrease ($p<0.05$). V_{Ao} and V_{PV} also increased after glucose load, with no change in V_{HA} (Table 3). Baseline TNF-a levels were detectable, but low, and were similar in all groups.

Haemodynamic and Metabolic Parameters After Endotoxin

EDTX-induced hypotension was comparable in the three groups over the 180-min observation time, but with different flow patterns (Table 2). In fed

Table 1. Glycogen content (equivalent glucose per g wet liver tissue weight) in four liver samples from fed rabbits and from fasting rabbits before and 30 min after the end of intra-portal infusion of 4 g glucose

	Glycogen
FED	404±99
FASTED	48±24
FASTED+GLC	142±40

Data expressed as mean±SE.

Table 2. Evolution of haemodynamic parameters in fed, 24-hours fasted and glucose-loaded rabbits before (T_0) and 180 min after iv EDTX.

		P_{Am} mmHg	V_{Ao} cm·s^{-1}	V_{PV} cm·s^{-1}	V_{HA} cm·s^{-1}
FED	T_0	85±3	16±1	16±4	26±2
	180 min	68±10[a]	9±4[a]	10±7[a]	28±6
FASTED	T_0	83±6	18±2	20±5	32±5
	180 min	66±7[a]	16±5	21±6	13±3[b]
FASTED+GLC	T_0	81±3	18±2	15±3	16±3
	180 min	61±10[a]	7±3[a]	9±4[a]	8±5[a]

Mean arterial pressure (P_{AM}), ascending aorta (V_{Ao}), portal vein (V_{PV}) and hepatic artery (V_{AH}) blood flow velocities, expressed as mean±SE. [a] $p<0.05$, [b] $p<0.01$ (intragroup ANOVA).

Table 3. Haemodynamic and metabolic parameters in pre (baseline) and post (Glc load) glucose infusion conditions (4 g glucose intraportally) in 24-hours fasted rabbits.

	P_{Am} mmHg	V_{Ao} cm·s^{-1}	V_{PV} cm·s^{-1}	V_{HA} cm·s^{-1}	pH	$PaCO_2$ Torr	PaO_2 Torr	HCO_3^- mmol/l
Baseline ($n=10$)	81±3	18±2	15±3	16±3	7.36±0.02	35±2	469±18	21.6±0.9
Glc load ($n=10$)	84±2	21±2.0 [a]	23±5 [a]	7±3	7.31±0.01 [a]	41±2 [a]	395±28	20.5±0.8

Mean arterial pressure (P_{AM}), ascending aorta (V_{Ao}), portal vein (V_{PV}) and hepatic artery (V_{AH}) blood flow velocities, blood gas measurements (pH, $PaCO_2$, PaO_2, HCO_3^-), expressed as mean±SE. [a] $p<0.05$, [b] $p<0.01$ (paired t-test).

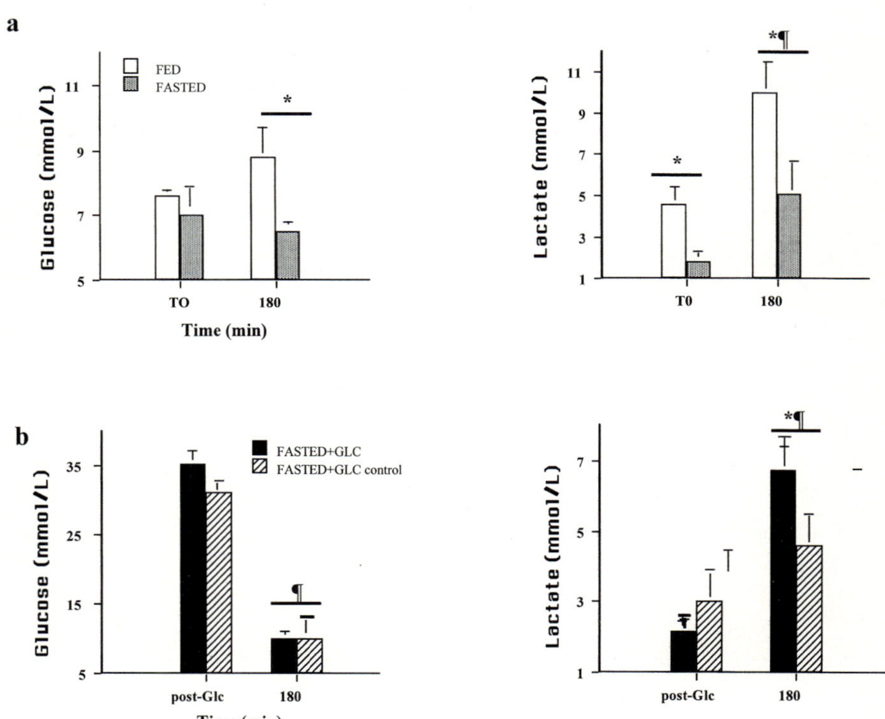

Fig. 1. a Plasma glucose and lactate concentrations in fed rabbits (*white bars*) and in rabbits after a 24-h fast (*shaded bars*) after i.v. endotoxin (EDTX) injection (T_0). **b** Plasma glucose and lactate kinetics after an intraportal glucose load (*Glc*, 2 g/kg) in fasting rabbits with i.v EDTX (*black bars*) or saline (*hatched bars*) injected after the glucose load. *$p<0.05$ for the intergroup comparison, ¶ for intragroup comparison, two-way analysis of variance (ANOVA) for repeated measures; data expressed as mean±SE

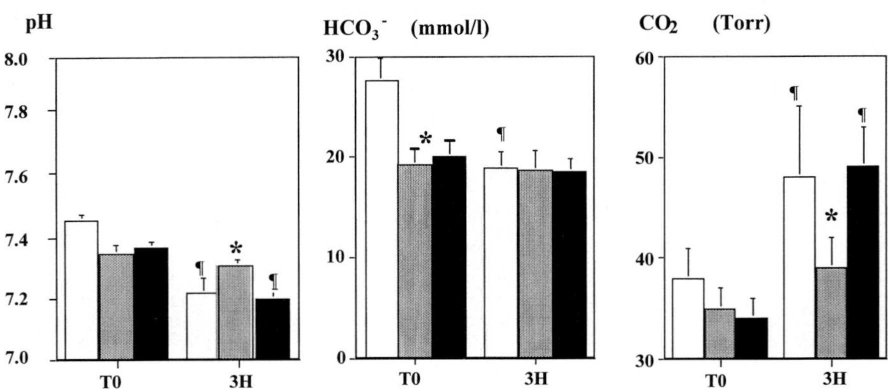

Fig. 2. Arterial acid–base status in endotoxin (EDTX)-treated rabbits in fed (*white bars*), fasting (*shaded bars*) and glucose-loaded, fasting (*black bars*) groups. *$p<0.05$ for the intergroup comparison, ¶ for intragroup comparison, two-way analysis of variance (ANOVA) for repeated measures, data expressed as mean±SE

animals, V_{Ao} decreased after EDTX injection (by 40%, $p<0.05$). V_{PV} decreased in parallel with systemic flow (by 40%, $p<0.05$) after EDTX, while V_{HA} remained unchanged. In fasting animals, EDTX did not change V_{Ao}. In these animals, compared to the fed group, systemic flow was significantly higher in relation to systemic vasodilatation. V_{PV} did not change, whereas the decrease in V_{HA} (by 70%, $p<0.05$) was more pronounced than in the fed group, accounting for local vasoconstriction.

Metabolic variables were also modified after EDTX injection. Both glucose and lactate levels increased in fed animals (Fig. 1a), with a pH and HCO_3^- decrease associated with hypercapnia (Fig. 2). In fasting animals, glucose, pH and HCO_3^- remained unchanged compared to t_0, with only a slight increase in the lactate level ($p<0.05$). Glucose and lactate variations significantly differed from the fed animals (Fig. 1a).

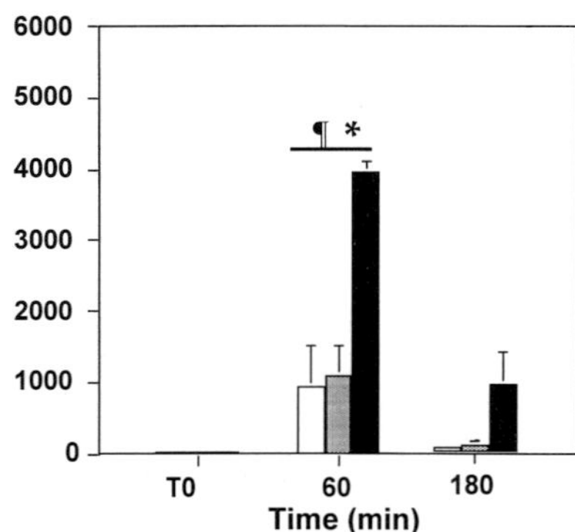

Fig. 3. Arterial kinetics of plasma tumour necrosis factor (TNF-a) in endotoxin (EDTX)-treated rabbits in fed (*white bars*), fasting (*shaded bars*) and glucose-loaded, fasting (*black bars*) groups. *$p<0.05$ for intergroup comparison, ¶ for intragroup comparison, two-way analysis of variance (ANOVA) for repeated measures, data expressed as mean±SE

In glucose-loaded, fasting animals, EDTX challenge induced different patterns when compared with the other two groups. For a similar hypotension, V_{Ao} decreased from control (by 60%, $p<0.05$) to a greater extent than in the fed group ($p<0.05$). However, V_{PV} and V_{HA} had comparable trends with relation to the fed group. Figure 1b shows the plasma glucose and lactate concentration variations in glucose-loaded, fasting animals with and without EDTX. Surprisingly, EDTX injection did not influence the course of glycaemia, whereas the lactate level reached was higher after EDTX ($p<0.01$). In the glucose-loaded, fasting group, EDTX induced a pH decrease, with hypercapnia and lactate production, but with no change in bicarbonate (Fig. 2). Acidosis corresponded to both metabolic and respiratory mechanisms. After 180 min, these modifications were similar to those observed in the fed group.

Inflammation After Endotoxin Injection

In the fed and fasting groups, EDTX injection induced a similar increase in arterial plasma TNF-α levels, which peaked 1 h after EDTX injection and decreased to control values after 3 h. Compared with the two other groups, the glucose-loaded, fasting group had similar pre-EDTX levels. One of the most striking results concerned the dramatic increase in TNF-α levels after EDTX in the glucose-loaded, fasting group (Fig. 3). The peak value was fourfold greater ($p<0.01$) than those observed in the other groups, with a similar concentration decay.

Arterial NOx concentrations (Table 4) were lower in the normally fed group compared with the other two groups. However, after EDTX, NOx increased significantly over time in the fed group (by 300%, $p<0.05$). In the other two groups, nitrite levels did not change after EDTX and were comparable in all groups after 3 h.

Table 4. Evolution plasma NOx (nitrite/nitrate) in fed, fasted and glucose-loaded fasted rabbits after iv EDTX.

NOx (μmol/l)	FED	FASTED	FASTED+GLC
T_0	15±2	32±13	54±12 [a]
60 min	23±20	34±13	45±8
120 min	41±19	54±22	49±6
180 min	46±14 [b]	38±16	44±8

[a] $p<0.05$ (intergroup comparison, compared to FED). [b] $p<0.05$ (intragroup comparsion, compared to T_0), data expressed as mean±SE.

Discussion

To our knowledge, no study has evaluated the impact of glucose availability simultaneously on the haemodynamic, metabolic and inflammatory response to EDTX. According to the literature, modification of glucose metabolism after EDTX challenge seems to have haemodynamic [8] or immune consequences [17, 19].

Because of the long surgical preparation before EDTX injection, control values may have been influenced by surgical stress. This non-specific inflammation may account for the detectable plasma TNF-α and for the elevated lactate levels without metabolic acidosis or hypoxia seen in fed animals. This hyperlactataemia was not observed in fasting animals, a duration which appeared sufficient to deplete liver glycogen stores. Consequently, a relative energy deficit may have stimulated firstly gluconeogenesis with lactate uptake, and secondly fatty acid oxidation, leading to an overproduction of ketone bodies. The observed metabolic acidosis with normal lactate concentrations in fasting animals before EDTX is consistent with this hypothesis.

The protocol conditions should also be discussed. As previously shown [18], glucose loading in fasting animals led to rapid glycogen formation (within 30 min). This synthesis was accompanied by an increased glycolysis, as suggested by the increase in lactate and $PaCO_2$ (at a constant ventilation). The portal route for glucose infusion was chosen in order to be able to control the quantity delivered and to mimic oral glucose loading [1, 6], while avoiding gastrointestinal secretion in association with digestion and absorption. The fasting may affect other substrates as well as glucose, such as proteins and lipids, potentially interfering with the observed results. Since the data obtained in the glucose-loaded, fasting group resembled those observed in the fed group, we concluded that at least glucose metabolism modifications can explain the results. Metabolic data such as $PaCO_2$, lactate and glycogen kinetics were in accordance with this concept.

Haemodynamic Modifications

EDTX injection induced similar hypotension in the three groups. However, in fed animals a low cardiac output and systemic vasoconstriction were observed with a decreased portal flow in parallel with systemic flow, as previously shown [22]. The trend for hepatic arterial blood flow was similar in fed and glucose-loaded animals; the level at the end of the protocol was close to the pre-EDTX level or was slightly decreased in glucose-loaded animals, in accordance with the arterial buffer response concept [15]. In fasting animals, hepatic arterial blood flow was not maintained, but decreased after EDTX. Vasoconstriction may result from a direct or indirect effect of EDTX secondary to oxygen-reactive species (ORS), NO deficit or a particular response of this vascular bed.

Elevated plasma glucose concentration may play a role, based on ex vivo experimental studies performed on non-septic animals [5]. Glucose impairs endothelium-dependent relaxation in vitro in relation with synthesis of vasoconstrictor prostanoids after glucose exposure [25] and with the increased synthesis of endothelial ORS [26]. In the three different study conditions, it is tempting to relate glycaemia and systemic conductance. In the fasting group, the absence of hyperglycaemia after EDTX was associated with systemic vasodilatation, whereas in the two other groups, particularly in glucose-loaded animals, glycaemia was elevated after EDTX, in parallel with the amplitude of systemic vasoconstriction.

It has also been shown that high extracellular glucose concentration impairs the endothelial release of NO, which partly mediates the alteration of vascular smooth muscle cell Na^+-K^+ ATPase pump, responsible for impairment in vascular relaxation [12]. NOx concentration may reflect the balance between production and consumption of NO. A deficit in NO release during hyperglycaemic situations was not observed in the present study, since plasma NOx levels did not differ between the three groups after EDTX. Nevertheless, it should be noted that the fed group had a baseline concentration of NOx significantly lower than the fasting groups. This may result from interaction with ORS [14]. One can speculate that the fed animals produced higher levels of ORS in association with glucose metabolism activation due to surgical preparation and stress. Such an ORS production may consume NO, explaining a lower control value of NOx. Further studies are needed to test this hypothesis.

Other aspects need to be discussed in the light of haemodynamic data. TNF-a is a well-known cytokine involved in vascular hypocontractility [27, 29]. In the present study, the highest peak observed in glucose-loaded animals was accompanied by the lowest vascular conductance. This supports the idea that other factors can predominate over the TNF-a-induced depression of vascular contraction. Among these, $PaCO_2$ and pH may play an important role. In normally fed and glucose-loaded animals, arterial pH decreased in association with both lactic acidosis and hypercapnia. Hypercapnia may have partly induced systemic vasoconstriction [10]. This is substantiated by the metabolic acidosis with normocapnia observed in fasting animals after EDTX which was accompanied by systemic vasodilatation.

Inflammatory Response

Classic kinetics of arterial TNF-a concentration were observed in our model. The most striking result concerned the large increase in TNF-a release in fasting animals receiving intraportal glucose before EDTX injection. TNF-a peaked at fourfold higher levels compared with the other groups. Comparison of the TNF-a response observed in the fasting groups allowed us to interpret this activation of TNF-a release in connection with glucose metabolism. After glucose loading, hepatic glycogen stores have been partially restored and plasma levels of glucose after EDTX were higher than in the fasting situation. The improvement in glucose availability might be responsible for the amplitude of the immuno-inflammatory response. It has been shown that, during sepsis, tissue glucose uptake is enhanced, especially in immuno-competent organs or cells. Among these, macrophages and granulocytes increase their glucose incorporation ex vivo after stimulation by EDTX [17]. Moreover, the amplitude of IL-1β release ex vivo by human EDTX-stimulated monocytes is positively correlated with the glucose concentration in the culture medium [19]. Such concepts seem to be verified in vivo.

No differences between arterial, portal and hepatic vein TNF-α levels have been observed after EDTX (data not shown). This may result from the marked stimulation of the whole immune system, which could mask the specific contribution of the liver, an organ which both produces [7] and clears TNF-α [9].

Metabolic Response

EDTX-induced variations in plasma glucose and lactate levels and $PaCO_2$ should be analysed together because of their metabolic link. In the fed group following EDTX, plasma glucose and lactate increased in parallel with hypercapnia, leading to a mixed blood acidosis. In the fasting group, plasma glucose levels and $PaCO_2$ did not change after EDTX, whereas lactate levels varied in a similar range to that in the fed group. This difference appeared to be mainly related to glucose, since the glucose-loaded, fasting group had similar patterns to fed animals. According to previous studies [23], glycogenolysis in the fed group would been activated after EDTX, leading to overproduction of lactate and CO_2. This implies a sufficient intra-hepatocyte storage of glycogen. As observed after a 24-h fast, hepatic glycogen was largely decreased, thus reducing the efficiency of glycogenolysis. The observation of a stable and quite normal glucose concentration and $PaCO_2$ after EDTX in the fasting group further supports the hypothesis of decreased glycogenolysis. The mechanism of hyperlactataemia needs further investigation to differentiate lactate overproduction and impairment of captation and metabolism.

As far as glucose metabolism during sepsis is concerned, in addition to hyperglycogenolysis, a relative insulin resistance impairing peripheral glucose uptake has been shown [23]. Interestingly, kinetics of plasma glucose level after intraportal glucose load did not differ between endotoxaemic and normal animals. This suggests that, in this model at an early phase of EDTX shock, the peripheral glucose uptake is not influenced by EDTX. However, lactate kinetics differed in these two situations, suggesting a modification in metabolic pathways. During the first 60 min, plasma lactate levels increased similarly in both groups. Thereafter, lactate levels only further increased in endotoxaemic animals, suggesting additional mechanisms for lactate increase after EDTX. The initial phase may result from activation of glycolysis in relation to substrate overload. The difference in the second phase might be related to mechanisms induced by EDTX injection, such as overstimulation of glycogenolysis (although glycaemia and PaCO$_2$ were identical in both groups) and impairment of lactate uptake.

In conclusion, the glucose status influences the haemodynamic, inflammatory and metabolic response to EDTX. Such a concept may have clinical implications, and the possibility of providing nutritional support in septic patients and of modulating their inflammatory response should be discussed.

Acknowledgements. We are indebted to Dr. Catherine Bernard (Paris, France) for TNF-α measurements and helpful comments; Jean-Louis Beaudeux (Paris, France), who made possible various biochemical measurements; Prof. Xavier Leverve and Prof. Christophe Pison (Grenoble, France) for glycogen determination in the liver and their encouraging discussion; and Hiroshi Ohshima (Lyon, France) for nitrite measurements. This work was supported by the Institutional Grant Programme of the Paris VII University, the *Direction de la Recherche et de l'Enseignement Doctoral* 1990–1995 and the *Assistance Publique-Hôpitaux de Paris*, contract 1990–1994. Dr. Losser received the Young Investigator Award 1994 from the Société Française d'Anesthésie–Réanimation for part of these data.

References

1. Adkins A, Myers SR, Hendrick G, Stevenson RW, Williams PE, Cherrington AD (1987) Importance of the route of intravenous glucose delivery to hepatic glucose balance in the conscious dog. J Clin Invest 79:557–565
2. Bagby GJ, Lang CH, Spitzer JJ (1993) Cytokine modulation of glucose metabolism. In: Schlag G, Redl H (eds) Pathophysiology of shock, sepsis, and organ failure. Springer, Berlin Heidelberg New York, pp 593–608
3. Bernard C, Szekely B, Philip Y, Wollman E, Payen D, Tedgui A (1992) Activated macrophages depress the contractility of rabbit carotids via an L-arginine/nitric oxide-dependent effect or mechanism. Connection with amplified cytokine release. J Clin Invest 89:851–860
4. Billiar T, Curran R, Ferrari F, Williams D, Simmons R (1990) Kupffer cell: hepatocyte cocultures release nitric oxide in response to bacterial endotoxin. J Surg Res 48:349–353
5. Cohen RD, Woods HF (1993) Lactic acidosis revisited. Diabetes 32:181–191
6. Cywes R, Greig PD, Sanabria JR, Clavien P-A, Levy GA, Harvey PRC, Strasberg SM (1992) Effect of intraportal glucose infusion on hepatic glycogen content and degradation, and outcome of liver transplantation. Ann Surg 216:235–247
7. Decker K (1990) Biologically active products of stimulated liver macrophages (Kupffer cells). Eur J Biochem 192:245–261
8. Esahili AH, Boïja PO, Ljungqvist O, Rubio C, Ware J (1991) Twenty-four hour fasting increases endotoxin lethality in the rat. Eur J Surg 157:89–95
9. Ferraiolo BL, Moore JA, Crase D, Gribling P, Wilking H, Baughman RA (1988) Pharmacokinetics and tissue distribution of recombinant human tumor necrosis factor-α in mice. Drug Metab Dispos 162:270–275
10. Gelman S, Ernst EA (1977) Role of pH, PCO$_2$, and O$_2$ content of portal blood in hepatic circulatory autoregulation. Am J Physiol 233:E255-E262
11. Green LC, Wagner DA, Glogowski J, Skipper PL, Wishnok S, Tannenbaum SR (1982) Analysis of nitrate, nitrite, and [^{15}N]nitrate in biological fluids. Anal Biochem 126:131–137
12. Gupta S, Sussman I, McArthur CS, Tornheim K, Cohen RA, Ruderman NB (1992) Endothelium-dependent inhibition of Na$^+$-K$^+$ ATPase activity in rabbit aorta by hyperglycemia. Possible role of endothelium-derived nitric oxide. J Clin Invest 90:727–732
13. Hartley CJ, Cole JS (1974) An ultrasonic pulsed Doppler system for measuring blood flow in small vessels. J Appl Physiol 37:626

14. Kubes P (1993) Ischemia-reperfusion in feline small intestine: a role for nitric oxide. Am J Physiol 264 (Gastrointest Liver Physiol 27):G143-G149

15. Lautt WW (1983) Relationship between hepatic blood flow and overall metabolism: the hepatic arterial buffer response. Fed Proc 42:1662–1666

16. Lavanchy N, Martin J, Rossi A (1984) Glycogen metabolism: a ^{13}C-NMR study on the isolated perfused rat heart. FEBS Lett 178:1–4S

17. Meszaros K, Bojta J, Bautista AP, Lang CH, Spitzer JJ (1991) Glucose utilization by Kupffer cells, endothelial cells, and granulocytes in endotoxemic rat liver. Am J Physiol 260:G7–G12

18. Mullany CJ, Wolfe RR, Burke JF (1980) The fate of a glucose infusion in fasting and fed guinea pigs: glucose oxidation rates and the distribution of glucose in liver, muscle and adipose tissue. J Surg Res 29:116–125

19. Orlinska U, Newton RC (1993) Role of glucose in interleukin-1β production by lipopolysaccharide-activated human monocytes. J Cell Physiol 157:201–208

20. Pastor CM, Billiar TR, Losser MR, Payen DM (1995) Liver injury during sepsis. J Crit Care 104:1–17

21. Pastor CM, Losser MR, Payen D (1995) Nitric oxide donors prevents hepatic and systemic perfusion decrease induced by endotoxin in anesthetized rabbits. Hepatology 22:1547–1553

22. Pastor CM, Payen D (1994) Effect of modifying nitric oxide pathway on liver circulation in a rabbit endotoxin shock model. Shock 23:1–7

23. Sacco-Gibson NA., Filkins JP (1989) Macrophages, monokines, and the metabolic pathophysiolgy of septic shock. Prog Clin Biol Res 286:203–218

24. Shangraw RE, Jahoor F, Miyoshi H, Neff WA, Stuart CA, Herndon DN, Wolfe RR (1989) Differentiation between septic and postburn insulin resistance. Metabolism 3810:983–989

25. Tesfamariam B, Brown ML, Deykin D, Cohen RA (1990) Elevated glucose promotes generation of endothelium-derived vasoconstrictor prostanoids in rabbit aorta. J Clin Invest 85:929–932

26. Tesfamariam B, Cohen RA (1992) Free radicals mediate endothelial cell dysfunction caused by elevated glucose. Am J Physiol 263:H321-H326

27. Tracey KJ, Beutler B, Lowry SF, Merryweather J, Wolpe S, Milsark IW, Hariri RJ, Fahey TJ III, Zentalla A, Albert JD, Shires GT, Cerami A (1986) Shock and tissue injury induced by recombinant human cachectin. Science 234:470–474

28. Tredget EE, Ming Yu Y, Zhong S, Burini R, Okusawa S, Gelfand JA, Dinarello CA, Young VR, Burke JF (1988) Role of interleukin 1 and tumor necrosis factor on energy metabolism in rabbits. Am J Physiol 255 (Endocrinol Metab 18):E760–E768

29. Vicaut E, Hou X, Payen D, Bousseau A, Tedgui A (1991) Acute effects of tumor necrosis factor on the microcirculation in rat cremaster muscle. J Clin Invest 87:1537–1540

30. Wu Y, Chen J, Ohshima H, Pignatelli B, Boreham J, Li J, Campbell TC, Peto R, Bartisch H (1993) Geographic association between urinary excretion of N-nitroso compounds and oesophageal cancer mortality in China. Int J Cancer 54:713–719

Neutrophil Elastase, C-Reactive Protein and Platelet Count After Severe Multiple Trauma Indicate the Risk for Late Multiple Organ Failure Following Secondary Operations

C. Waydhas, D. Nast-Kolb, R. Zettl, A. Trupka, L. Schweiberer, and M. Jochum

Abstract

The objective of this study was to determine the role of both specific and non-specific indicators of the inflammatory response in their ability to indicate the risk of patients with severe multiple injuries of developing late organ failure following secondary operations. In a prospective study of 106 severely injured patients (mean injury severity score, ISS, 40.6) who underwent secondary operations (>3 days after trauma), we compared the level of preoperative inflammation with the sequelae of surgical trauma. The interventions included facial reconstructions, osteosynthesis of the pelvic girdle, long bones and spine, and others. Group 1 comprised 40 patients (38%) who developed respiratory, renal and/or hepatic failure within 2 days after the operation or whose pre-existing organ dysfunction worsened by more than 20% from baseline. The remaining 66 patients (62%) with an uneventful recovery formed group 2. The preoperative levels of neutrophil elastase (92.2 vs. 61.3 ng/dl), C-reactive protein (12.4 vs. 7.6 mg/dl) and platelet count (118 vs. 236 1000/µl) were significantly more abnormal in the patients in group 1. The pO_2 to FiO_2 ratio was also somewhat lower in group 1 patients (305.5 vs. 351), whereas other parameters, e.g. cathepsin B, interleukin (IL)-6, blood pressure, heart rate, bilirubin, creatinine, urinary output, lactate, pH and coagulation, were not able to differentiate preoperatively between groups 1 and 2. An increased state of inflammation (neutrophil elastase, >85 ng/ml; C-reactive protein, >11 mg/dl; platelet count, <180 000/µl) predicted postoperative organ failure with an accuracy of 79% (sensitivity, 73%; specificity, 83%). In conclusion, secondary operations may act as a second hit and precipitate late multiple organ dysfunction syndrome if they are done in multi-trauma patients while the patients still have an increased level of post-traumatic inflammation. If the levels of neutrophil elastase and C-reactive protein are elevated and the platelet count is low, a further delay of surgery or a change of method might be beneficial.

Introduction

Primary stabilization of major fractures in patients who have sustained multiple injuries is an important component of early trauma management. However, immediate intramedullary nailing of femural shaft fractures may not be indicated in certain patterns of injuries, such as concomitant pulmonary contusion [1]. There is no general agreement about whether pelvic instabilities should be repaired on the day of trauma or at some time later, unless there life-threatening haemorrhage occurs [2–4]. It is recommended that patients with injuries to the spine should be operated on only after they have recovered from the sequelae of the primary insult if they are neurologically stable [5]. Many other types of injuries do not require an urgent operation and are postponed until a later period in the post-traumatic course.

However, it has been shown that secondary surgery of major orthopaedic injuries might be associated with increased morbidity and mortality rates [6, 7]. The consequences of surgical trauma are thought to be similar to those of accidental blunt trauma, e.g. disruption of tissue, blood loss, pain, interruption of normal food and fluid uptake [8]. Alterations in homeostasis [8], hormone levels [9], the immune response [10–12], neutrophil elastase levels [13, 14], C-reactive protein, IL-6 and other cytokines [15–17] have been shown to occur after trauma as well as postoperatively and reflect a dose-dependent response, with larger operations causing larger changes. Thus (secondary) operations may be viewed as an additional insult imposed on subjects that are already hampered by the sequelae of the initial accident. Therefore, we conducted a study in order to determine the role of surgical procedures as secondary inflammatory insults in the development of late multiple organ dysfunction syndrome in patients with multiple trauma; we also evaluated both laboratory and clinical indicators of the inflammatory response in their ability to indicate the risk of severely injured patients of developing organ failure following secondary operations.

Materials and Methods

The investigation was planned as a prospective cohort study. Patients were included in the study only if all of the following criteria were met: (a) less than 6 h between the accident and admission to our emergency department, (b) age between 16 and 70 years, (c) severe injuries (abbreviated injury scale, AIS, ≥ 3) of more than one region (head, thorax, abdomen, pelvic girdle and extremities) or more than two major fractures, and (d) survival for at least 3 days.

Throughout the patients' stay in the surgical intensive care unit, blood for routine laboratory and special biochemical measurements was drawn every morning (at 7a.m.). Documentation of the patients' cardiopulmonary status and a clinical assessment was also done at this time.

After primary stabilization of the patients' vital signs in the emergency room, our treatment protocol called for immediate operative treatment of all life- and organ-threatening injuries. Fractures of the femoral shaft were not immediately stabilized by intramedullary nailing if the patient was unstable despite aggressive resuscitation or if there was a concomitant severe thoracic injury (AIS, ≥ 3). Fractures of the pelvic ring and the spine were managed by delayed surgery unless urgent intervention was necessary, e.g. severe bleeding or progressive neurologic deficit, respectively. Secondary (elective) operations were performed only if the patient was judged to be in a stable condition by the intensivist, the anaesthetist and the trauma surgeon alike. None of the patients presented with severe organ dysfunction, and their cardiopulmonary and coagulation parameters were under control.

The following definitions of organ dysfunction were used:
- *Respiratory failure:* requirement of mechanical ventilation plus a pO_2 to FiO_2 ratio of less than 280 or a positive end-expiratory pressure above 8 cmH_2O for more than 48 h.
- *Liver failure:* bilirubin levels of more than 51 µmol/l for more than 48 h.
- *Renal failure:* serum creatinine of more than 177 µmol/l for more than 48 h.
- *Postoperative organ failure:* organ failure (respiratory, liver or renal failure) beginning within 48 h of the operation or deterioration of a pre-existing organ dysfunction by more than 20% from baseline within 48 h after the operation and of least 2 days' duration. The cut-off value (20%) was intended to be large enough to rule out non-specific or minor variations of organ function parameters.

White blood count, platelet count, creatinine, bilirubin, lactate, partial thromboplastin time and prothrombin time were measured by routine clinical chemistry. The anti-thrombin III-inhibiting capacity was determined by a chromogenic substrate test (Kabi-Vitrum, Moelndal, Sweden). C-reactive protein was measured by radial immunodiffusion on liquid chromatography (LC)-partigen plates (Behringwerke, Marburg, Germany). Neopterin was quantified by means of a radio-immunoassay (Henning, Berlin, Germany); for the measurement of polymorphonuclear elastase-a_1–proteinase inhibitor complex (called neutrophil elastase for the sake of simplicity), we used an enzyme immunoassay (Merck, Darmstadt, Germany). The actual version of this test refers to a different standard than the former test. Thus the values of the new version presented here are one third of the values of the version that was used in former publications [18, 19]. IL-6 was determined using the IL-6 human enzyme-linked immunosorbent assay (ELISA) system (Amersham, Braunschweig, Germany), a quantitative sandwich enzyme immunoassay with a specific monoclonal antibody. Cathepsin B was measured by a fluorometric test developed by Machleidt et al. [45]. During dilution, inactive cathepsin B in plasma will be released from its complex with inhibitor and high molecular weight kininogen. The free enzyme cleaves Z-Phe-Arg-methyl-cumarinamide under formation of amino-methylcumarin, whose fluorescence is determined at 460 nm.

Statistical analysis was done with the chi-squared test or the non-parametric Wilcoxon-Mann-Whitney U test. A difference was considered significant with $p<0.05$ in the former and $p<0.001$ in the latter test. Receiver operator characteristics (ROC) analysis was used for determining cut-off points [20–22]. Sensitivity and specificity and the true positive and negative ratios (Bayes' theorem) were calculated by standard formulas [21].

The study was performed according to the guidelines of the ethics committee of the Ludwig-Maximilian University of Munich.

Results

A total of 133 patients with multiple injuries were included in the study. Their mean ISS was 40.6 (range, 13–75). Of these patients, 120 underwent a total of 376 operations during their stay at our institution. There were 67 urgent surgical procedures (within 24 h after trauma), 29 early operations (24–72 h after trauma) and 280 secondary surgical interventions (later than 72 h after trauma). Of the latter, 106 procedures were performed during the observation period while the patients were still in the intensive care unit. These 106 secondary operations constitute the study population. They comprised the following: osteosynthesis of the tibial shaft ($n=7$), the femur ($n=22$), the pelvic girdle ($n=13$) and the spine ($n=4$), reconstructions of fractures of the facial bones or the frontal basal skull ($n=19$); and other interventions ($n=41$), such as smaller osteosynthesis, tracheostomies and plastic surgery.

Forty of these patients developed postoperative pulmonary, renal and/or hepatic failure (group 1), whereas 66 subjects had an uneventful recovery (group 2), resulting in a 38% incidence of postoperative organ failure. There were no differences between patients in groups 1 and 2 with respect to age, sex, injury severity or day of surgery (Table 1). The distribution of injuries in different body regions was also similar in the two patient groups. The severity of injuries to the head and neck tended to be somewhat lower in group 1, and to the thorax somewhat lower in group 2. However, the differences between the two groups did not reach significance ($p>0.1$). Postoperative organ failure was observed following stabilization of femur and pelvic girdle fractures in 17 of 35 patients and after other types of procedures in 23 of 71 patients. Intra-operative data concerning blood loss, hypotension, volume balance, duration of surgery and contamination are presented in Table 2. There were no significant differences for any of these between patients with and without postoperative organ failure.

Further influencing factors on the course of recovery or the development of organ failure might be infections of various kinds. For a definition of pneumonia, catheter-related, urinary tract and other infections, we used the guidelines issued by the Center of Disease Control. The incidence of infections at the time of surgery was evenly distributed in the two patient groups without differences in subjects with or without postoperative organ failure. The data are detailed in Table 3.

Table 1. Data of patients with and without postoperative organ failure with operative interventions later than 72 h after trauma

	Group 1 (with OF)	Group 2 (without OF)	p value
Operations (n)	40	66	NS
Age (years)			
Median	31.5	28	NS
Lower/upper quartiles	22–52.5	24–27	NS
Sex			
Male (n)	29	56	NS
Female (n)	11	10	NS
Day of surgery			
Median	7	8	NS
Lower/upper quartiles	5–7.5	6–12	NS
Severity score			
Median	36	41.5	NS
Lower/upper quartiles	29–47.5	30–50	NS
AIS head/neck[a]	2.5±1.9	3.2±1.9	NS
AIS thorax[a]	2.1±1.7	1.6±1.7	NS
AIS abdomen[a]	1.8±2.0	1.9±2.0	NS
AIS skeletal[a]	3.7±1.2	3.5±1.2	NS
AIS general[a]	1.0±0.7	1.2±0.6	NS

OF, postoperative organ failure; AIS, abbreviated injury scale; NS, not significant.
[a] Average±SD.

The preoperative values of the clinical and biochemical parameters followed in this study from patients with and without postoperative organ dysfunction are presented in Table 4. The levels before surgery of C-reactive protein and neutrophil elastase were significantly higher and platelet count was significantly lower in patients that developed postoperative organ failure compared to subjects with an uneventful course after the surgical intervention. The PO_2 to FiO_2 ratio was also significantly lower in group 1 patients. However, the absolute difference between groups was relatively small, and the median pO_2 to FiO_2 ratio of group 1 and 2 was within normal limits (>280). Parameters of the cellular activation (cathepsin B, neopterin, IL-6) and of the humoral coagulation system (prothrombin time, partial thromboplastin time, anti-thrombin III) were similar in the two groups. No preoperative differences between the groups were found for indicators of the circulatory function (systolic blood pressure, central venous pressure, heart rate, pH), renal function (serum creatinine level, urinary output), hepatic function (serum bilirubin), or other indicators.

For those four factors that differentiated significantly between the two outcome groups, an ROC analysis was performed. The cut-off values resulting in

Table 2. Intra-operative data from 40 patients with and 66 subjects without postoperative organ failure

	Group 1 (with OF)	Group 2 (without OF)	p value
Blood loss (ml)			
Median	650	500	NS
Lower/upper quartiles	200–1400	150–700	NS
Systolic blood pressure <90 mmHg			
Patients (n)	3	4	NS
Percentage of group (%)	7.5	6.1	NS
Positive fluid balance (ml)			
Median	2150	1950	NS
Lower/upper quartiles	1030–4900	1150–3250	NS
Duration of sugery (min)			
Median	160	155	NS
Lower/upper quartiles	110–330	88–230	NS
Contamination of operative site[a]			
Patients (n)	13	25	NS
Percentage of group (%)	32.5	37.8	NS

OF, postoperative organ failure; NS, not significant.

[a] Contamination includes surgery on open fractures, frontal basal skull fractures or other contaminated areas.

Table 3. Incidence of infections at the time of surgery in 40 patients with and 66 patients without postoperative organ failure

State of infection at surgery[a]	Group 1 (with OF)		Group 2 (without OF)		p value
	(n)	(%)	(n)	(%)	
Ongoing infection	8	20.0	14	21.2	NS
Infection just beginning	10	25.0	21	31.8	NS
No infection	22	55.0	31	47.0	NS

OF, postoperative organ failure; NS, not significant.

[a] Infection includes pneumonia and catheter-related and urinary tract infections. An ongoing infection was assumed if the criteria for infection were met at least 2 days before surgery; the infection was thought to be just beginning if the criteria were met between 1 day before and 1 day after surgery. All other patients were free of infection.

the most accurate prediction of the postoperative course were 11.0 mg/dl for C-reactive protein, 85 ng/ml for neutrophil elastase, 180 000/µl for the platelet count and 280 for the pO_2 to FiO_2 ratio. The prognostic accuracies are shown in Table 5. They were highest for C-reactive protein (75%) followed by platelet count (71%), neutrophil elastase (70%) and pO_2 to FiO_2 ratio (68%). The combination of the three indicators of the inflammatory response yielded an accuracy of 79% if at least two of them were in the pathologic range. An abnormal or

Table 4. Preoperative values in patients with postoperative organ failure and in patients without complications that were operated on later than 72 h after trauma

	Group 1 (with OF; n=40)		Group 2 (without OF; n=66)		p value[b]
	Median	Quartiles[a]	Median	Quartiles[a]	
C-reactive protein (mg/dl)	12.4	9.6–17.6	7.6	4.4–10.8	<0.001
Lactate (mmol/l)	1.4	1.2–1.8	1.2	1.0–1.5	NS
Neopterin (nmol/l)	20.0	13.5–32.0	16.1	9.6–22.2	NS
Cathepsin B (U/ml)	87.5	69.1–108.9	93.5	67.1–116.8	NS
IL-6 (pg/ml)[c]	49	18–160	26	14–42	NS
Neutrophil elastase (ng/ml)	92.2	68.5–132.7	61.3	46.3–86.7	<0.001
Anti-thrombin III (% of normal)	83	68.5–94	96.5	84–112	NS
Platelet count (1000/µl)	118	92.5–186.5	236.5	162–374	<0.001
pO_2/FiO_2 ratio	305.5	263.5–357.5	351	316–409	<0.001
Creatinine (µmol/l)	70.7	61.9–97.2	70.7	61.9–88.4	NS
Bilirubin (µmol/l)	46.9	30.8–85.5	25.6	18.8–56.4	NS
White blood count (1000/µl)	12	9–17	14.5	10–19	NS
Systolic blood pressure (Torr)	140	130–150	130	120–140	NS
Central venous pressure (Torr)	10	5–13	7	4–12	NS
Partial thromboplastin time (s)	33	30–37	31	29–35	NS
Prothrombin time (% of normal)	89	81–95	88.5	81–97	NS
pH	7.43	7.39–7.45	7.43	7.41–7.45	NS
Heart rate (1/min)	119.5	105–123.5	105	90–122	NS
Urinary output (ml/24 h)	3100	2200–4420	2800	2250–3200	NS

IL, interleukin; OF, postoperative organ failure; NS, not significant.
[a] Lower and upper quartiles.
[b] Wilcoxon-Mann-Whitney U test.
[c] $n=18$ (group 1) vs. n=17 (group 2).

"pathologic" preoperative test result, e.g. two pathologic parameters, increased the probability of postoperative organ failure from 38% (incidence) to 73% (true positive ratio), whereas in the case of a negative test result, an uneventful course could be expected in 83% (true negative ratio).

Despite an overall accuracy of nearly 80% in the prediction of the operative risk, several patients were incorrectly classified. We hypothesized that a low preoperative inflammatory activity (baseline values on the "normal" side of

Table 5. Prognostic accuracy of C-reactive protein, platelet count and neutrophil elastase and of their combination in predicting postoperative organ failure in patients operated on later than 72 h after trauma

	Sensitivity (%)	Specificity (%)	True positive ratio (%)	True negative ratio (%)	Accuracy (%)
C-reactive protein[a]	65	79	65	79	75
Platelet count[b]	73	70	59	81	71
Neutrophil elastase[c]	63	74	60	77	70
At least *one* parameter in the pathologic range	95	58	50	93	62
At least *two* parameters in the pathologic range	73	83	73	83	79
All *three* parameters in the pathologic range	33	97	87	70	73

[a] Cut-off value, >11 mg/dl.
[b] Cut-off value, <180 000 µl.
[c] Cut-off value, >85 ng/ml.

the cut-off values) required a greater increase in the inflammatory response due to the surgical trauma (i.e. a major operation) to result in organ failure, whereas the additional effect of a minor intervention might not be detrimental even in face of high inflammatory baseline activity. Indeed, 79% of patients classified as being "false negative" (postoperative organ failure despite low indicators of inflammation) underwent major operative procedures, such as pelvic girdle and femur osteosynthesis. Conversely, 71% of interventions performed in those subjects that had an uneventful course despite a high preoperative inflammatory activity (classified as "false positive") were considered to be "minor".

Discussion

The post-traumatic multiple organ failure syndrome appears to follow a biphasic pattern with early (non-septic) and late (septic) organ failure [23]. This concept has been confirmed by other observations [19, 24–27]. It is hypothesized that early organ failure is caused by the initial post-traumatic inflammatory response ("one-hit" theory). The high accuracy in predicting outcome even on admission to hospital with the help of parameters such as lactate and base excess [28] and other indicators of the inflammatory response [18] favours this concept. However, much evidence is accumulating that late organ failure may be precipitated by a secondary insult ("two-hit" theory) [27, 29, 30]. This is usually thought to be uncontrolled infection or sepsis [27, 31, 32], mainly from pneumonia but also from other sites of infection [19, 25, 31, 33].

Our data indicate that surgery performed in the post-traumatic period may also act as a second hit and cause late organ failure; after 38% of secondary surgical interventions in severely injured patients, a deterioration of organ function was observed. There was a close relationship between surgery and the onset of organ failure, with the deterioration of function parameters starting within a period of 48 h after the operation in all of these subjects. Although a simultaneous additional insult as the cause for the organ failure cannot be ruled out with definite certainty in every single patient, this close correlation suggests a direct effect of surgery on the patients' course. Infections were observed at the time of surgery in a considerable percentage of patients, but their incidence was similar in patients that did not develop postoperative organ failure and in group 1 subjects. Therefore, our results appeared not to be hampered by an uneven distribution of infections. Furthermore, all subjects were in a stable condition before surgery and were not operated on during a phase of deteriorating respiratory, renal or hepatic function. The duration of postoperative organ failure was required to be at least 2 days in order to avoid transient minor changes in the pO_2 to FiO_2 ratio, creatinine and bilirubin being mistaken for organ failure.

Analysis of the patients' condition revealed a markedly increased state of inflammation (as indicated by C-reactive protein, neutrophil elastase and platelet count) before surgery in those individuals that consecutively developed organ failure, whereas subjects with an uneventful postoperative course had a low level of inflammation. The role of C-reactive protein, neutrophil elastase and platelet count in indicating the severity of the post-traumatic inflammatory response has been confirmed in many investigations [18, 19, 24, 34–36]. Thus our data suggest that severely injured patients with a persisting state of inflammation have an increased risk of developing postoperative complications when operated on at that time, despite the fact that their condition was stable with respect to coagulation, circulation and other organ functions.

The incidence of postoperative organ failure, however, is not only determined by the compensatory resources of the patient at the time of the operation, but also by the surgical trauma itself and its consequent disturbance of homeostasis [9, 37, 38]. The magnitude of the surgical trauma, as indicated by blood loss, intra-operative hypotension, fluid balance and duration of surgery, was evenly distributed between patients with and without postoperative organ failure and appeared not to have affected the relationship between the preoperative state of inflammation and outcome.

In the interrelationship between pre-existing and supervening lesions, mediators of the inflammatory response may play a crucial role. If we assume that the surgical trauma results in an inflammatory response [9, 15–17, 38] that adds to the pre-existing disturbance, it may be hypothesized that major operations, e.g. osteosynthesis of the pelvic girdle, may lead to postoperative complications even with a relatively low preoperative inflammatory activity, whereas smaller surgical procedures, e.g. facial reconstructions, will not result in organ failure despite a moderately disturbed baseline situation. Indeed, patients that have been rated "false-negative", i.e. patients with less abnormal markers of systemic inflammation but with postoperative organ failure, usually underwent major operations. Conversely, subjects with considerable inflammatory activity, but no postoperative organ dysfunction (rated "false positive") underwent minor operations in the majority of cases (71%).

From a clinical point of view, the data presented suggest that indicators [24, 26] of the inflammatory response such as C-reactive protein, neutrophil elastase, platelet count and respiratory function parameters, e.g. the pO_2 to FiO_2 ratio, may predict the risk of patients with multiple injuries of developing organ failure after secondary operations. In our hands, the combination of the three indicators of inflammation was the most useful in assessing outcome and allowed 79% accuracy in predicting postoperative organ failure in patients with severe injuries. We are not aware of any communications which refer to the role of platelet count and neutrophil elastase in this context, but Christou et al. [39] evaluated the relationship of preoperative C-reactive protein levels with outcome. In their study, the concentrations of C-reactive protein did not differ between survivors and non-survivors. However, in contrast to our severely traumatized patients, they investigated patients before elective abdominal surgery, with mean C-reactive protein levels of 1.6 and 1.7 mg/dl in the two outcome groups, which indicates no significant inflammatory activity before the operation.

The potential of C-reactive protein, neutrophil elastase and platelet count to predict the operative risk in patients with multiple injuries has to be compared with other known risk indicators. Well-known risk factors such as old age [39, 40], pre-existing cardiac disease [40] or chronically decreased respiratory function [37] are of little value, since the prevalence of these conditions is fairly low in a population of severely traumatized young patients. While the classification by the American Society of Anesthesiologists (ASA) [41] has described the general increased risk of this group of patients, it is not useful for the assessment of an individual subject in this setting. The clinical judgement of a physician experienced in trauma care may correctly estimate a patient's condition and his or her tolerance of surgical trauma. To our knowledge, there are, however, no communications available as to the clinical evaluation of the preoperative risk of critically ill trauma patients. Clinical judgement in this setting seems to be difficult and not very reliable. This is documented by the fact that we observed an incidence of postoperative organ failure of 38%, although a careful assessment by surgeons, anaesthetists and intensivists had taken place preoperatively and all of the patients had been deemed to be operable. The prognostic index presented by Shoemaker et al. [42], which accounts for 35 cardiorespiratory parameters, anticipated the outcome of surgical high-risk patients with a 94% accuracy. However, this analysis included measurements that were taken postoperatively and therefore cannot be used to estimate the risk preoperatively. In addition, easy to measure parameters, such as blood pressure, heart rate, central venous pressure and pH, were of relatively little prognostic relevance in their study [42, 43]. The poor role of these parameters in preoperative risk assessment was confirmed by our findings. Moreover, preoperative prothrombin time, partial thromboplastin time and lactate did not show any relevant prognostic potential in our study either. The first two of these parameters are primary targets for therapeutic intervention and are usually kept within the normal range in critically ill patients. The normal lactate levels (which are comparable in the two postoperative outcome groups) can be explained by close preoperative monitoring and immediate treatment of abberations that rendered substantial anaerobic metabolic situations unlikely.

Preoperative serum creatinine concentrations and urinary output were not different in patients with and without postoperative organ failure. Although bilirubin levels tended to be higher in patients with a complicated postoperative course, a sufficiently reliable distinction was not possible due to a considerable overlap between the groups. However, our data suggest that respiratory function parameters such as the pO_2 to FiO_2 ratio may predict the risk of secondary operations in severely injured patients at a certain point in time. Since trauma to the chest appears to be an independent risk factor for the development of post-traumatic respiratory failure [44], subjects with chest trauma have an increased probability of developing impaired respiratory function. The tendency towards more severe chest trauma in our patients with organ failure, although not significant, might thus be partially responsible for the observation that there was a significantly lower pO_2 to FiO_2 ratio in this group preoperatively. A predictive role of preoperative oxygen tension in arterial blood has already been observed by Savino and DelGuerico [43] in elderly high-risk patients. The cut-off value in their study was close to a pO_2 of 50 Torr at room air (FiO_2, 0.21), which corresponds to a pO_2 to FiO_2 ratio of 238. This somewhat lower cut-off point can be explained by the physiologically lower pO_2 in their elderly patients as compared to the population in our study. However, in our investigation, the median pO_2 to FiO_2 ratios were within a more or less normal range in both groups, and the absolute differences between the groups were comparatively small.

Thus a large number of classic criteria, predictors and indicators were of little value in our study in assessing the postoperative risk of severely injured patients. However, indicators of the inflammatory response (and of respiratory function) showed marked preoperative differences between patients with and without postoperative organ failure. This may allow for more reliable timing of secondary surgical procedures after severe trauma.

We conclude that secondary operations (>72 h after trauma) may act as a "second hit" in severely injured patients and may trigger postoperative organ failure. Subjects that are still in a state of increased post-traumatic inflammation (despite stable organ function) and/or undergo major surgery appear to be particularly susceptible to surgical trauma. Indicators of the inflammatory response (C-reactive protein, neutrophil elastase, platelet count) might help to identify patients at risk. Future investigations are needed to show whether postponing surgery until inflammation has subsided or the use of less invasive surgical techniques will decrease the rate of postoperative organ failure in the post-traumatic patient.

Acknowledgement. We would like to thank Bettina Vock, Susann Waydhas and Irene Schneider for their excellent assistance in carrying out this study and in analysing the results. Grants were provided by the Schutzkommission beim Bundesminister des Inneren, Bonn (ZS 8–122–42 project 5.9/85) and by the Sonderforschungsbereich SFB 207 (project G5), University of Munich.

References

1. Pape HC, Auf'm'Kolk M, Paffrath T et al (1993) Primary intramedullary femur fixation in multiple trauma patients with associated lung contusion – a cause of posttraumatic ARDS? J Trauma 34:540
2. Burgess AR, Mandelbaum BR (1987) Acute orthopedic injuries. In: Siegel JH (ed) Trauma. Emergency surgery and critical care. Churchill Livingston, New York, pp 1049–1074
3. Leenen LPH, Van der Werken C, Schoots F et al (1993) Internal fixation of open unstable pelvic fractures. J Trauma 35:220
4. Tile M (1987) Fractures of the pelvis. In: Schatzker J, Tile M (eds) The rationale of operative fracture care. Springer, Berlin, Heidelberg New York, pp 37–44
5. Marion D, Clifton G (1991) Injury to the vertebrae and spine. In: Moore EE, Mattox KL, Feliciano DV (eds) Trauma. Appleton and Lange, Norwalk, pp 261–275
6. Bone LB, Johnson KD, Weigelt J et al (1989) Early versus delayed stabilization of femoral fractures. J Bone Joint Surg 71:336
7. Seibel R, LaDuca J, Hassett JM et al (1985) Blunt multiple trauma (ISS36), femur traction, and the pulmonary failure-septic state. Ann Surg 202:283
8. Wilmore DW (1991) Homeostasis. Bodily changes in trauma and surgery. In: Sabiston DC (ed) Textbook of surgery. Saunders, Philadelphia, pp 19–33
9. Chernow B, Alexander HR, Smallridge RC et al (1987) Hormonal responses to graded surgical stress. Arch Intern Med 147:1273
10. Christou NV, Superina R, Broadhead M et al (1982) Postoperative depression of host resistance: determinants and effect of peripheral protein-sparing therapy. Surgery 92:786
11. Lennard TWJ, Shenton BK, Borzotta A et al (1985) The influence of surgical operations on components of the human immune system. Br J Surg 72:771
12. McLoughlin GA, Wu AV, Saporoschetz I et al (1979) Correlation between anergy and a circulating immunosuppressive factor following major surgical trauma. Ann Surg 190:297
13. Duswald KH, Jochum M, Schramm W et al (1985) Released granulocytic elastase: an indicator of pathobiochemical alterations in septicemia after abdominal surgery. Surgery 98:892
14. Cohen JR, Dietzek A, Tyras D et al (1989) Leukocyte and serum elastase in response to elective surgical trauma. J Cardiovasc Surg 30:817
15. Pullicino EA, Carli F, Poole S et al (1990) The relationship between the circulating concentrations of interleukin 6, tumor necrosis factor and the acute phase response to elective surgery and accidental injury. Lymphokine Res 9:231
16. Baigrie RJ, Lamont PM, Dallman M et al (1991) The release of interleukin-1beta (IL-1) precedes that of interleukin 6 in patients undergoing major surgery. Lymph Cytokine Res 10:253
17. Cruickshank AM, Fraser WD, Burns HJG et al (1990) Response of serum interleukin-6 in patients undergoing elective surgery of varying severity. Clin Sci 79:161
18. Nast-Kolb D, Waydhas C, Jochum M et al (1992) Biochemical factors as an objective parameter in assessing the severity and prognosis in polytrauma patients. Unfallchirurg 95:59
19. Waydhas C, Nast-Kolb D, Jochum M et al (1992) Inflammatory mediators, infection, sepsis, and multiorgan failure after severe trauma. Arch Surg 127:460
20. Begg CB (1987) Biases in the assessment of diagnostic tests. Stat Med 6:411
21. McNeil BJ, Keeler E, Adelstein SJ (1975) Primer on certain elements of medical decision making. N Engl J Med 293:21
22. Metz CE (1978) Basic principles of ROC analysis. Semin Nucl Med 4:283
23. Faist E, Baue EA, Dittmer H et al (1983) Multiple organ failure in polytrauma patients. J Trauma 23:775
24. Goris RJA, te Boekhorst TPA, Nuytinck JKS et al (1985) Multiple-organ failure. Generalized autodestructive inflammation? Arch Surg 120:1109

25. Sauaia A, Moore FA., Moore EE et al (1993) Pneumonia: cause or symptom of postinjury multiple organ failure? Am J Surg 166:606
26. Schlag G, Redl H, Hallström (1991) The cell in shock: the origin of multiple organ failure. Resuscitation 21:137
27. Barton R, Cerra FB (1989) The hypermetabolism multiple organ failure syndrome. Chest 96:1153
28. Siegel JH, Rivkind AI, Dalal S et al (1990) Early physiologic predictors of injury severity and death in blunt multiple trauma. Arch Surg 125:498
29. Anderson BO, Harken AH (1990) Multiple organ failure: inflammatory priming and activation sequences promote autogenous tissue injury. J Trauma 30:S44
30. Moore FA, Moore EE, Read RA (1993) Postinjury multiple organ failure: role of extrathoracic injury and sepsis in adult respiratory distress syndrome. New Horizons 1:538
31. Fry DE, Pearlstein L, Fulton RL et al (1980) Multiple system organ failure. The role of uncontrolled infection. Arch Surg 115:136
32. Eiseman B, Baert R, Norton L (1977) Multiple organ failure. Surg Gynecol Obstet 144:323
33. Meakins JL (1990) Etiology of multiple organ failure. J Trauma 30:S165
34. Nuytinck JKS, Goris RJA, Redl H et al (1986) Posttraumatic complications and inflammatory mediators. Arch Surg 121:886
35. Pacher R, Redl H, Frass M et al (1989) Relationship between neopterin and granulocyte elastase plasma levels and the severity of multiple organ failure. Crit Care Med 17:221
36. Rivkind AI, Siegel JH, Guadalupi P et al (1989) Sequential patterns of eicosanoid, platelet, and neutrophil interactions in the evolution of the fulminant post-traumatic adult respiratory distress syndrome. Ann Surg 210:355
37. Vodinh J, Bonnet F, Touboul C et al (1989) Risk factors of postoperative pulmonary complications after vascular surgery. Surgery 105:360
38. Waydhas C, Nast-Kolb D, Kick M et al (1993) Operative trauma of spine surgery in patients with multiple injuries. Unfallchirurg 96:62
39. Christou NV, Tellado-Rodriguez J, Chartrand L et al (1989) Estimating mortality risk in preoperative patients using immunologic, nutritional, and acute-phase response variables. Ann Surg 210:69
40. Goldman L, Caldera DL, Nussbaum SR et al (1977) Multifactorial index of cardiac risk in noncardiac surgical procedures. N Engl J Med 297:845
41. Vacanti CJ, VanHouten RJ, Hill RC (1970) A statistical analysis of the relationship of physical status to postoperative mortality in 68,388 cases. Anesth Analg 49:564
42. Shoemaker WC, Appel PL, Bland R et al (1982) Clinical trial of an algorithm for outcome prediction in acute circulatory failure. Crit Care Med 10:390
43. Savino JA, DelGuerico LRM (1985) Preoperative assessment of high-risk surgical patients. Surg Clin North Am 65:763
44. Gaillard M, Herve C, Mandin L et al (1990) Mortality prognostic factors in chest injury. J Trauma 30:93
45. Assfalg-Machleidt I, Jochum M, Klaubert W et al (1988) Enzymatically active cathepsin B dissociating from its inhibitor complexes is elevated in blood plasma of patients with septic shock and some malignant tumors. Biol Chem Hoppe-Seyler 369:263

Monitoring of Serum Cytokeratin 18 in Patients with Burns

G.S. Bayer, S.E. Andert, W.A. Bauer, A.E. Werbal, and G. Meissl

Introduction

Cytokeratin 18 (Cyt 18) is a protein belonging to the family of epithelial intermediate filament proteins forming the cytoskeleton of epithelial tissues. The management of severely burned patients in the early period after injury is extremely difficult, and parameters reflecting the course of illness in these patients would be helpful in their treatment and in determining their prognosis. Accordingly, we evaluated the usefulness in monitoring severely burned patients of the following parameters: Cyt 18, C-reactive protein (CRP), the immunoglobulins IgG, IgM and IgA, the complement factors C3c and C4, albumin, haptoglobin (HAP), α_1-anti-trypsin (AAT), acid α_1-glyco-protein (AAG) and anti-thrombin III (AT III).

Materials and Methods

In a retrospective study, the sera of 12 severely burned patients, nine males and three females (age range, 14–89 years, mean, 50.5±35.5 years), were analysed. Four of the 12 patients died. Total body surface area (TBSA) was calculated using the Dubois formula. The injured skin extended from 15% to 65% 2nd degree+3rd degree TBSA (survivors, 15%–65% 2nd degree+3rd degree; non-survivors, 17%–35% 2nd degree+3rd degree). Daily blood sampling was begun immediately after admission of a patient and as long as a patient was monitored in the intensive care unit. Cyt 18, CRP, immunoglobulins and acute-phase proteins were analysed using automated immunometric methods.

Results

Table 1 compares the Cyt 18 and CRP results in the survivors and non-survivors. The mean serum levels of Cyt 18 ($p<0.0236$) and CRP ($p<0.0253$) were significantly higher in non-survivors than in survivors. Survivors never had Cyt 18 concentrations of more than 300 U/l for longer than 4 days. In con-

Table 1. Cytokeratin 18 (Cyt 18; ref. range 0–80 U/l) and C-reactive protein (CRP; ref. range 0–12 mg/l) levels in survivors and non-survivors

Group	Cyt 18 (U/l)[a]			CRP (mg/l)[b]		
	Median	Mean±SD	Peak	Median	Mean±SD	Peak
Survivors ($n=8$)	154	180±141	792	210	211±106	489
Non-survivors ($n=4$)	385	937±1438	7700	306	326±146	689

trast, non-survivors exhibited a steady increase in Cyt 18 serum levels, which were greater than 300 U/l for longer than 4 days and continued to increase until death. A maximum concentration of Cyt 18 of 7700 U/l was recorded in the non-survivor group. There was no correlation between the burned surface area and Cyt 18 levels (r, 0.1). Mean serum levels of all other measured parameters were not significantly different between the two groups.

Conclusions

Cyt 18 is one of 20 cytokeratin proteins which have been isolated from different epithelial tissues forming the cytoskeleton and which contribute to its cellular shape and structure. Cytokeratins are located within the cell and are known to be secreted into the systemic circulation. After thermal injury, large parts of the skin are destroyed and the body attempts to repair this damage by proliferation of keratinocytes, fibroblasts, smooth muscle cells and endothelial cells. This proliferation might lead to increased synthesis and release of Cyt 18 from these cells and may cause the significant increase in serum Cyt 18 levels. The Cyt 18 results from this study suggest that measurement of this parameter may be useful in predicting the outcome in heavily burned patients and may reflect the proliferation and differentiation of damaged cells and subsequent repair mechanisms after injury from burns.

Intermittent Bolus Dosing of Ceftazidime in Critically Ill Patients

R. J. Young, J. Lipman, T. Gin, G. D. Gomersall,
G. M. Joynt, and T. E. Oh

Introduction

The bactericidal activity of β-lactam antibodies is related entirely to the time that concentrations in tissue and serum exceed a certain threshold, and higher concentrations do not produce added efficacy. If antibiotic concentrations decrease to below this threshold, bacterial growth is resumed immediately [1]. Ceftazidime, a β-lactam antibiotic, is frequently used in critically ill patients, particularly for the treatment of *Pseudomonas aeruginosa* infections. The recommended dosing regimen is based on pharmacokinetic data obtained in healthy volunteers and may not be appropriate in the critically ill [2]. The aim of this study was to determine whether the current recommended regimen for ceftazidime maintains adequate serum concentrations for antibacterial efficacy in critically ill patients.

Methods

We administered ceftazidime at the maximum recommended dosage (2 g every 8 h intravenously) to ten intensive care patients with normal renal function. Plasma samples were taken at timed intervals over 8 h with a further trough sample taken on day 3. Ceftazidime concentrations were measured by high-performance liquid chromatography. Pharmacokinetic analysis was performed with MK MODEL (Biosoft, Cambridge, UK).

Results

Although the pharmacokinetic parameters for ceftazidime were similar to previously reported data in normal volunteers, there was large interpatient variability in drug concentrations. Three of the patients had plasma ceftazidime below the published minimal inhibitory concentration (MIC) of *Pseudomonas aeruginosa* of up to 8 µg/ml [3], and nine patients had concentrations below five times the MIC which has been recommended to ensure efficacy [1]. On day 3, trough ceftazidime concentrations were less than the MIC in four out of seven patients in whom measurements were made and less than five times the MIC in the remaining three. There was no clinical predictor of which patients would have low plasma concentrations.

Conclusions

Our results suggest that the recommended dosing regimen for ceftazidime may result in inadequate tissue concentrations and loss of bactericidal efficacy. This may be overcome by more frequent boluses or continuous infusion.

References

1. Mouton JW, den Hollander JG (1994) Killing of Pseudomonas aeruginosa during continuous and intermittent infusion of ceftazidime in an in vitro pharmacokinetic model. Antimicrob Agents Chemother 38:931–6
2. Rudy AC, Brater DC (1994) Pharmacokinetics. In: Chernow B (ed) The pharmacologic approach to the critically ill patient. Williams and Wilkins, Baltimore, pp 3–17
3. Scribner RK, Marks MI, Weber AH et al (1982) Activities of various β-lactams and aminoglycosides, alone and in combination, against isolates of Pseudomonas aeruginosa from patients with cystic fibrosis. Antimicrob Agents Chemother 21:939–43

Biochemical Prognostic Markers in Critically Ill Patients

P. Zivny, V. Cerny, L. Zabka, V. Palicka, and L. Pliskova

Introduction

The aim of the study was twofold. The first was to characterise the pattern of interleukin (IL)-6 and tumour necrosis factor (TNF)-α secretion in patients with trauma and in critically ill patients without trauma. The second aim was to relate this secretion to patient outcome.

Methods

The subjects in this study were 12 patients with trauma (seven survivors, five non-survivors) and 11 patients who were critically ill but without trauma (six survivors and five non-survivors). Blood samples were taken at 0, 12 and 24 h after admission to the intensive care unit. Cytokine levels were measured using enzyme-linked immunosorbent assays (ELISA).

Results

The TNF-α and IL-6 results from samples taken at 0, 12 and 24 h are presented in Table 1. The only significant differences between the groups of patients were for the TNF-α results, which were significantly higher in those patients with trauma who did not survive than in those trauma patients who recovered.

Conclusions

These results suggest that TNF-α may be a useful prognostic marker in patients who are critically ill due to multiple trauma.

Table 1. Levels of cytokines (mean±SEM) in survivors and non-survivors with and without trauma

Cytokine	Patient group	Time after admission		
		0 h	12 h	24 h
TNF-α (mg/l)	Trauma survivors	3.2±1.7	2.8±1.9	4.3±2.0
	Trauma non-survivors	17.9±7.2[*]	13.2±4.8[*]	17.6±5.5[*]
	Non-trauma survivors	13.5±2.2	11.5±2.5	12.5±4.2
	Non-trauma non-survivors	9.3±0.8	8.7±2.7	12.9±3.0
IL-6 (U/ml)	Trauma survivors	177±58	95±51	75±45
	Trauma non-survivors	238±73	148±46	154±57
	Non-trauma survivors	156±81	88±54	65±39
	Non-trauma non-survivors	117±68	150±76	157±94

TNF, tumour necrosis factor; IL, interleukin.

[*] $p < 0.05$.

Decreased L-Selectin Expression on Polymorphonuclear Leucocytes Following Dexamethasone Treatment: Another Possible Anti-Inflammatory Mechanism

D. Weisman, A. Tang, S. Granleese, S. F. Van Eeden, J. C. Hogg, and G. P. Bondy

Introduction

Inflammation of small airways is an important feature in the development of bronchopulmonary dysplasia (BPD) following hyaline membrane disease in premature babies. Dexamethasone is an effective treatment for BPD since it reduces lung inflammation through a poorly understood mechanism. The cell adhesion molecule L-selectin is essential for the initiation of recruitment of leucocytes to areas of inflammation [1, 2]. The purpose of this study was to determine the effect of dexamethasone on the expression of L-selectin on circulating polymorphonuclear leucocytes (PMN) and monocytes; these effects were measured in premature babies with BPD and in rabbits.

Methods

The patients is this study were 20 babies who received dexamethasone and 28 who were untreated. The effects of L-selectin on leucocytes and monocytes were measured as mean fluorescence intensity (MFI) using immunofluorescent flow cytometry. Intravascular cell activation was measured as changes in CD18 expression.

Similar measurements were carried out on five rabbits after treatment with 1 mg dexamethasone/kg per day, and these results were compared to those of three control rabbits.

Results

There were no significant differences in the gestational age, birth weight and sex between the two groups of babies, but the chronological age in the dexamethasone group was higher ($p<0.05$). In the dexamethasone-treated group, total white cell count and PMN count were higher ($p<0.001$), while L-selectin expression was lower on circulating PMN (5.67 ± 0.6 vs. 10.64 ± 0.7, $p<0.0001$) and on monocytes (7.85 ± 0.9 vs. 12.5 ± 0.8, $p=0.02$) than in the non-treated babies. There was no difference in the CD18 expression levels in the two groups, and L-selectin levels before starting dexamethasone and after it was discontinued were similar to the levels in the non-dexamethasone-treated group.

In rabbits treated with dexamethasone, there was a rise in PMN count 6 h after the first dose, with a subsequent decrease after 24 h; a 173% increase from baseline was observed after 72 h of treatment. L-selectin levels fell to 59% of baseline values after 24 h of treatment. There was no difference in the CD18 levels between the two groups, and studies of α-bromodeoxyuridine-labelled cells demonstrated that the leucocytosis produced by dexamethasone was related to mobilisation of cells from the bone marrow.

Conclusions

L-selectin is important for the recruitment of PMN to inflammatory foci. We suggest that one of the mechanisms by which dexamethasone reduces inflammation is by impairing the ability of leucocytes to migrate into inflamed tissues. In addition, studies are currently underway to determine the clinical utility of neutrophil L-selectin levels in monitoring the effect of dexamethasone therapy in patients with BPD.

References

1. Burton JL, Kehrli ME Jr, Kapil S et al (1995) Regulation of L-selectin and CD18 on bovine neutrophils by glucocorticoid effects of cortisol and dexamethasone. J Leukoc Biol 57:317–325
2. Mulligan MS, Miyasaka M, Tamatani T et al (1994) Requirements for L-selectin in neutrophil-mediated lung injury in rats. J Immunol 152(2):832–840

Thrombocytopaenia Associated with the Systemic Inflammatory Response Syndrome: Involvement of the Haemophagocytosis Process

B. Francois, F. Trinoreau, H. Gastinne, and V. Praloran

Introduction

Acute thrombocytopaenia is a common occurrence in critically ill patients; it carries a high mortality risk, but the causes are often unknown. The haemophagocytic syndrome has recently been described as a phagocytosis of bone marrow cells by patient-activated macrophages. Since intensive care patients diagnosed with thrombocytopaenia frequently exhibit a systemic inflammatory response syndrome (SIRS), which is characterised by high circulating cytokine levels, we conducted a prospective study to determine the incidence of the haemophagocytosis process (HP) and to determine whether SIRS and HP involve common mechanisms triggered by high circulating cytokine levels.

Methods

Over a 1-year period patients with an SIRS (according to Bone's criteria, with a platelet count of less than $100\,000/mm^3$ of undetermined aetiology) underwent a sternal marrow aspiration, and macrophage colony-stimulating factor (M-CSF) in serum was measured. Patients were subsequently divided into two groups according to the presence or absence of evidence of haematopoetic cell phagocytosis. Serum M-CSF levels of 59 normal subjects were measured during the same period and were used to define a reference range.

Results

Of 50 consecutive patients recruited into the study (mean age, 57±16 years), 32 exhibited an HP. The severity of acute illnesses on admission as assessed by the Acute Physiology and Chronic Health Evaluation (APACHE) II score was similar in the two groups (21.7±6 vs. 24.2±4, not significant). Table 1 shows the platelet count, organ dysfunction (as defined by the Odin model [1]), incidence of sepsis and M-CSF levels in the two groups.

Table 1. Platelet count, organ dysfunction, incidence of sepsis and levels of macrophage colony-stimulating factor (M-CSF) in patients with and without evidence of haematopoetic cell phagocytosis (mean±SD)

Patient group	Platelet count $(10^3/mm^3)$	Organ dysfunction (n)	Patients with sepsis (n)	M-CSF (U/ml)
With HP (n=32)	60.5±25	1.9±0.8	17	580±145
Without HP (n=18)	75.5±25	1.0±0.4	3	457±89
p value	0.05	0.0001	0.02	0.01

HP, Haemophagocytosis process.

Conclusions

An HP appears to be a frequent cause (64%) of unexplained thrombocytopaenia in intensive care patients suffering from SIRS, particularly when sepsis or shock is present. Haematopoetic cell phagocytosis in critically ill patients may be related to a higher circulating level of M-CSF. Better knowledge of cytokine production in the HP would improve the prognosis and management of patients with SIRS.

References

1. Fagon JY, Chastre J, Novara A et al (1993) Characterisation of intensive care unit patients using a model based on the presence or absence of organ dysfunctions and/or infection: the Odin model. Intensive Care Med 19:137–144

Use of Cortisol, Glucagon and Nitrogen Balance Measurements To Assess Stress Levels in Critically Ill Patients

C. Pichard, U. Kyle, N. Mensi, and R. Gaillard

Introduction

Muscle catabolism in response to stress commonly occurs in critically ill patients despite optimal nutritional support. Recent evidence indicates that recombinant human growth hormone (rhGH), despite its normal anabolic effects, does not reverse the catabolic status in highly stressed patients. Given the expense of recombinant hormone, it is necessary to identify those patients who are not highly stressed and who will benefit from this therapy. The aim of this study was to determine low (LS), medium (MS) and severe stress (SS) states on a clinical basis in intensive care patients and to validate this clinical judgement by objective metabolic measurements in order to select early those ICU patients who can potentially benefit from rhGH therapy.

Methods

Thirty-six consecutive intensive care patients were classified as LS, MS or SS by two experienced senior intensive care consultants using temperature, agitation, heart rate, arterial blood pressure, presence of infection, respiratory rate and exogenous catecholamines as indicators. Anabolic (insulin; insulin-like growth factor-1, IGF-1; GH) and catabolic (cortisol, glucagon) hormones together with nitrogen balance were determined for each patient within 8 h after admission to the intensive care unit. Biochemical and clinical data were compared by analysis of variance (ANOVA).

Results

The results of biochemical parameters for the various stress states are shown in Table 1.

Table 1. Biochemical parameters in the various stress states (mean±SE)

	Low stress	Medium stress	Severe stress	p value
Insulin (pmol/l)	40.9±6.4	59.3±9.9	80.3±28.3	NS
IGF-1 (mg/l)	79.7±6.7	67.4±5.4	58.1±8.7	NS
GH (ng/dl)	1.59±0.49	1.44±0.38	3.14±0.77	NS
Cortisol (nmol/l)	530±55	755±70	878±109	0.013
Glucagon (pg/ml)	123±40	163±27	319±64	0.009
N_2 balance[a] (g/day)	−4.2±1.2	−10.6±1.6	−8.1±2.2	0.037

IGF, insulin-like growth factor; GH, growth hormone; NS, not significant.

[a] Values given for nitrogen balance are the mean over 3 days.

Conclusions

The clinical stress states determined by intensive care physicians correlated
well with catabolic hormone levels and the nitrogen balance. This data suggests that measurement of these parameters can identify patients who are
more likely to benefit from adjuvant rhGH therapy. A prospective study of
rhGH therapy in mildly stressed intensive care patients is in progress.

Prognostic Implications from Measurement of Cytokines in Bronchoalveolar Lavage in Critically Ill Patients with Pneumonia

S. M. Samir, S. A. El-Shafee, A. Hatem, and S. Mokhtar

Introduction

Pneumonia is a frequent complication of critically ill patients and often leads to respiratory failure in patients whose immune system is compromised. The aim of this study was to evaluate protected bronchoalveolar lavage (PBAL) as a diagnostic procedure in patients with pneumonia and to evaluate the pattern of cytokine secretion in the lavage specimens.

Methods

Fibreoptic bronchoscopy was carried out in 38 patients diagnosed with pneumonia, 14 of which had ventilator-acquired disease, six with non-ventilator-but hospital-acquired disease and 18 with community-acquired disease. Control studies were carried out in 15 healthy subjects. Cultures were made on sputum, bronchoalveolar lavage and PBAL. In addition, cytology was carried out on specimens from PBAL, and tumour necrosis factor (TNF), interleukin-8 (IL-8) and interleukin-2 receptor (IL-2R) were measured. These parameters and complement were also measured in serum from the same patients. The Acute Physiological and Chronic Health Evaluation (APACHE) II score was estimated for each patient on admission and at discharge or death.

Results

The mortality rate in the 38 patients was 39%, and the APACHE II score was more than 20 in all patients who died. The PBAL procedure had a sensitivity of 73.7% and a specificity of 100%, with a positive predictive value of 100% and a negative predictive value of 60%. The results for cytokine and complement levels in serum and PBAL specimens are shown in Table 1.

Serum TNF was elevated in 29% of patients, while PBAL TNF was elevated in 76%; serum IL-8 was elevated in 42%, and PBAL IL-8 in 76% of patients; serum IL-2R was elevated in 60.5%, and PBAL IL-2R in 47.4% of patients. Serum complement was elevated in 92% of patients.

Table 1. Cytokine and complement levels in serum and protected bronchoalveolar lavage (PBAL) specimens (mean±SD)

	Source of pneumonia			Controls
	Ventilator acquired	Hospital acquired	Community acquired	
TNF serum	41±52	89.8±143.9	32±39.9	5.7±2.2
TNF PBAL	145.9±155.3	139.5±137	222.6±191.63	0
IL-8 Serum	227.6±419.4	836.5±1806	299±845	28.7±8.8
IL-8 PBAL	5050±4484	6160±4595	7043±4198	426±33.6
IL-2R serum	3577.6±2595.5	3925±2612.9	1908.4±1495.5	1350±150
IL-2R PBAL	385.5±7	194.3±196	124.4±160.6	50±10
Complement	221±87	242±86	245±76	113±7.8

TNF, Tumour necrosis factor; IL-8, interleukin-8; IL-2R, interleukin-2 receptor.

Conclusions

PBAL is more specific, but less sensitive than other methods of sampling. The APACHE II score was a good prognostic tool for the detection of high-risk patients and for prognostic follow-up.

Hypoxia – Ischaemia

Changes in Serum and Cerebrospinal Fluid Superoxide Dismutase and Neurone-Specific Enolase Following Acute Cerebral Ischaemia

A. Miller, B. Gross, H. Rawashdi, R. Almog, S. Honigman, M. Barak, and N. Gruener

Introduction

The release of inflammatory cytokines and free radicals is believed to be one of the events associated with experimental cerebral ischaemia. Superoxide dismutase (SOD) is a key enzyme in anti-oxidative protection, and neurone-specific enolase (NSE) has been proposed as a marker for neuronal injury. The aim of this study was firstly to examine the changes in blood and cerebrospinal fluid (CSF) levels of SOD and NSE following acute stroke, and secondly to relate these changes to infarct size and patient outcome.

Methods

CSF and serum SOD and NSE were measured on days 1–7 after the onset of acute cerebral ischaemia in 43 patients with large hemispheric infarction and 48 patients with lacunar infarcts. Control samples were obtained from 17 patients with lower back pain. Copper/zinc SOD was measured by competitive enzyme-linked immunosorbent assay (ELISA) using antibodies against recombinant SOD raised in rabbits. NSE was measured with a sandwich immunoassay which contains monoclonal and polyclonal antibodies to NSE.

Results

The results showed a rise in serum and CSF NSE that reached a peak 48 h after the onset of ischaemia and remained high for 7 days. NSE levels were directly correlated to infarct size, as determined by computed tomography. Levels of SOD rose within the first 24 h, reached a peak at 48 h and declined towards day 7. Increases in SOD were larger in the patients with lacunar infarcts. There was a trend of association between elevated levels of both NSE and SOD at 48 h and the mortality rate at 2 months after the onset of cerebral ischaemia.

Conclusions

These results suggest that NSE and SOD are distinctly regulated after cerebral ischaemia. NSE levels may be a guide to infarct size, while both serum NSE and SOD levels may represent prognostic markers after stroke. Further biochemical studies are required to elucidate the mechanisms underlying the pathophysiology of cerebral ischaemia. Such information may be useful in identifying high- and low-risk patients and for identifying future anti-ischaemic treatment strategies.

Human Polymorphonuclear Leucocyte Metabolism and Lipoperoxidation During Adult Respiratory Distress Syndrome

G. Lefevre, F. Brunet, M. Roch-Arveiller, J.-F. Dhainaut, and J. P. Giroud

Introduction

The purpose of this study was to investigate circulating polymorphonuclear leucocyte (PMNL) oxidative metabolism and lipid peroxidation in patients with adult respiratory distress syndrome (ARDS) who were treated with low-frequency, positive-pressure ventilation with extracorporeal carbon dioxide removal.

Methods

PMNL from patients with ARDS were incubated either with phosphate buffered saline (PBS), with serum from ARDS patients or with normal serum. Oxidative metabolism was assessed by chemiluminescence, while PMNL proteases were assessed by determining circulating levels of complexed elastase. Oxidative stress status was determined by assaying plasma lipid peroxidases, as judged by malondialdehyde concentration (MDA) and erythrocyte glutathione peroxidase activity (E-GPx). The results in surviving and non-surviving patients were compared with matched controls, and the data was analysed using the Mann-Whitney test; $p \leq 0.05$ was considered significant.

Results

The chemiluminescence of PMNL from ARDS patients was significantly enhanced when compared to control PMNL ($p < 0.001$). Preincubation of PMNL from ARDS patients with sera from either controls or ARDS patients resulted in a significant decrease in chemiluminescence ($p < 0.05$). Results for E-GPx, plasma MDA and elastase concentrations in surviving and non-surviving patients are shown in Table 1.

There was a significant correlation between chemiluminescence of PMNL from ARDS patients and elastase levels (r, 0.82; $p < 0.001$) and between MDA concentration and the Injury Severity Score score [1] (r, 0.46; $p = 0.056$).

Table 1. Erythrocyte glutathione peroxidase activity (E-GPx) and plasma malondialdehyde (MDA) and elastase concentrations in survivors and non-survivors (mean±SD)

	Controls ($n=15$)	All patients ($n=15$)	Survivors ($n=7$)	Non-survivors ($n=8$)
MDA (μmol/l)	0.34±0.14	0.54±0.26*	0.64±0.32*	0.45±0.16
E-GPx (IU/gHb)	45±8	48±12	56±8**	40±11***
Elastase (μg/l)	22±10	172±121****	131±103*	208±129****

* $p<0.05$ vs. controls; ** $p<0.01$ vs. controls; *** $p<0.01$ vs. survivors; **** $p<0.001$ vs. controls.

Conclusions

Our results demonstrate that oxygen metabolism and elastase levels of circulating PMNL from ARDS patients are significantly enhanced. In spite of the increase in lipid peroxidation of ARDS sera, no correlation could be demonstrated between PMNL functions and plasma peroxidation. Our results confirm that PMNL from ARDS patients are primed either by bacterial products or cytokines released during the course of the acute phase of the illness, but free radicals produced by the PMNL cells seem to be only one of the events responsible for the extent of lipid peroxidation.

References

1. Knaus WA, Draper EA, Wagner DP et al (1985) Prognosis in acute organ-system failure. Ann Surg 202:685–693

Cardiology – Haemodynamics

Left Ventricular Assist Device Powered by a Balloon Counterpulsation Console

M. Calderon

Abstract

Mechanical circulatory support systems have been shown to give adequate clinical results in patients with severe heart failure, but most existing devices are only available in a few centres because of their high cost. To meet the needs of ventricular assist devices (VAD) in Mexico, we designed a model to study the feasibility of using a conventional counterpulsation console as a drive module (Mexi-Cor programme).

We built a sac-type artificial left ventricle, with a non-thrombogenic polyurethane 50-cc chamber and two 21 mm prosthetic disc valves (inflow and outflow). In vitro tests showed adequate driving pressures and an output of 4 l at a fixed rate of 80 bpm. Experimental animal studies demonstrated full haemodynamic support of the excluded left ventricle during 8 hour acute experiments. The device can be placed in a paracorporeal position or implanted in the abdomen in an extra-peritoneal fashion.

Our results demonstrate that counterpulsation consoles can drive ventricular assist devices (VAD), hence reducing complexity and costs. We believe that these type of devices may be suitable for future therapy in patients requiring short-term mechanical cardiac support. Intensive multi-centre research is required to further investigate this treatment.

Introduction

In recent years, a better understanding of the pathophysiology of cardiac diseases as well as advances in diagnostic techniques, operative procedures and myocardial preservation have resulted in significant improvements in the outcome of cardiac surgery. These advances are resulting in a worldwide trend of cardiologists and surgeons treating more seriously ill patients.

Cardiogenic shock with low output state, which follows either myocardial infarction or cardiac surgery or is the result of chronic heart failure, has a mortality rate of almost 100% if the condition is not responsive to the use of balloon counterpulsation and maximal pharmacological therapy [1]. Considerable progress has been made during the past two decades in the development of mechanical circulatory support devices, ranging from short-term partial support systems to devices which can completely support the circulation for months [2]. The use of VAD is based on the premise that ventricular function may be able to recover provided that there is a period of rest for the injured myocardium [3] and that systemic circulation is maintained at the same time. Where there is no cardiac recovery, the device provides high-quality circulatory support to allow the patient to undergo a successful heart transplantation [4].

Despite the satisfactory clinical results achieved with the use of the available ventricular support systems, either as a bridge to recovery or to cardiac transplantation, their high cost means that their use is limited to a few centres worldwide and to only small series of patients. With the exception of centrifugal pumps, which are indicated for very short ventricular support, the remainder of the commercially available VAD range in cost from US$ 60000 to US$ 300000 for the drive consoles and from $ 7000 to $ 45000 for the prosthetic ventricles (according to product information for the year 1995 from Thermo Cardiosystems Inc., Woburn, MA; Thotatec Laboratories Corp., Berkeley, CA; Baxter-Novacor Division, Oakland, CA; Abiomed Cardiovascular Inc., Danvers, MA and Fehling Medical AG, Berlin).

Due to the urgent need for this kind of therapy in Mexico and the limited funds available, we established a research programme named Mexi-Cor ("Mexican heart") with the aim of developing a simple, economic and effective method of circulatory support for the failing heart.

We hypothesised that this could be achieved by the development of a simple, sac-type, pneumatic, prosthetic ventricle which could be driven by a conventional intra-aortic counterpulsation balloon console. This rationale was based on the fact that most local and international cardiac facilities have existing facilities and expertise in counterpulsation therapy. The aim of this project was therefore to provide a device that could be driven by any brand of console and supplied in different volumes so as to be suitable for both paediatric and adult patients.

Materials and Methods

A pneumatically driven, sac-type VAD was designed and built with a non-thrombogenic, biocompatible, polyurethane 50 cc chamber. In order to make it unidirectional, the inflow and outflow tracts have 21 mm disc prosthetic mechanical valves (Fig. 1). The device was designed to support left ventricular function in a parallel fashion by placing the inflow cannula in the left atrium (behind the interatrial groove or via the left atrial appendage), and the outflow cannula is anastomosed to the ascending aorta. Both cannulae were customised in our research laboratory. The atrial cannula is a wire-reinforced, 36-Fr cannula with a 45° angle, and the aortic cannula is a wire-reinforced, straight, 36-Fr cannula with a 12 mm preclotted Dacron graft at the distal end (Fig. 2). The

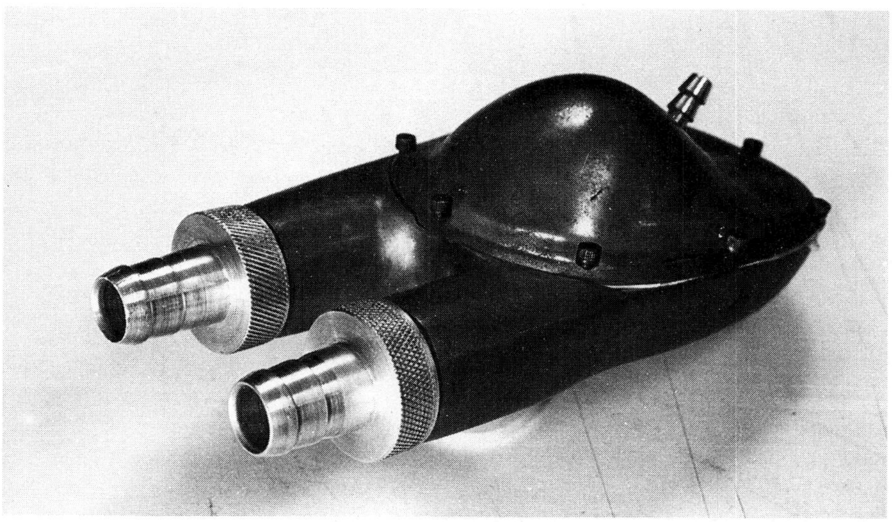

Fig. 1. Mexi-cor – paracorporeal, pulsatile left ventricular assist device

device could be utilised either in the paracorporeal (subcostal) position or implanted in the abdomen outside the peritoneal cavity.

In Vitro Test

The 50 cc sac-type VAD was tested in a mock circulatory loop. A Model 95 Datascope (Datascope Corporation, Montvale, NJ) balloon counterpulsation console was used to drive the pump (with vacuum) at a fixed rate of 80 bpm for periods of up to 30 days.

In Vivo Test

Eight healthy male mongrel dogs, weighing 40–48 kg, were utilised for 8 hour acute experiments. All animal experimentation was done according to the *Institutional Animal Care and Use Committee Guidebook* [5]. After induction of general anaesthesia and placement of invasive monitoring lines, a median sternotomy was made. The heart was exposed and heparin (3 mg/kg) was administered. Without the use of cardiopulmonary bypass, the inflow and outflow cannulae were placed in the left atrium and ascending aorta, respectively. The VAD was primed with lactated Ringer's solution and connected to the cannulae. The blood pump was driven by the counterpulsation console synchronised with the animal's electrocardiogram at pump rates of 1:1 and 1:2. The experiments lasted 8 h with continuous monitoring of haemodynamic parameters, arterial blood gases and urine output. During the last two experiments, the left anterior descending coronary artery was ligated.

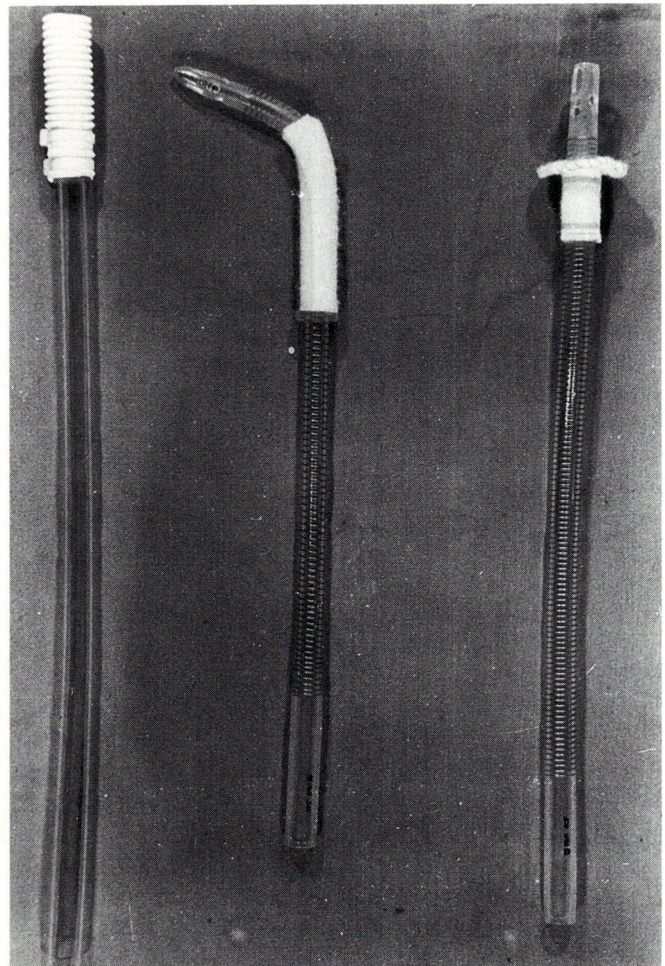

Fig. 2. Customised cannulae for vascular assist device implantation (aortic, atrial, ventricular)

Results

In Vitro Test

At a fixed rate of 80 bpm, with the use of the console's vacuum system, a filling pressure of 16 mmHg and 100 mmHg of afterload, the assist device provided an output (flow rate) of approximately 4 l/min (Fig. 3). During the tests, there was no evidence of material or prosthetic valve dysfunction for up to 30 days after insertion of the prosthesis.

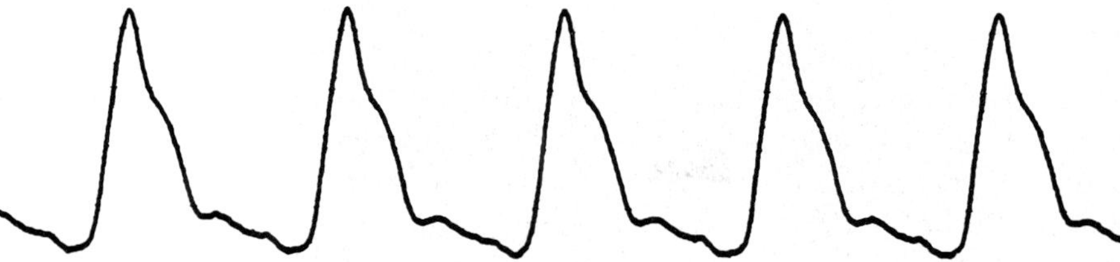

Fig. 3. Vascular assist device pressure trace during in vitro test in mock circulatory loop. Heart rate, 80 bpm; mean arterial pressure, 51 mmHg; systole/diastole, 110/25

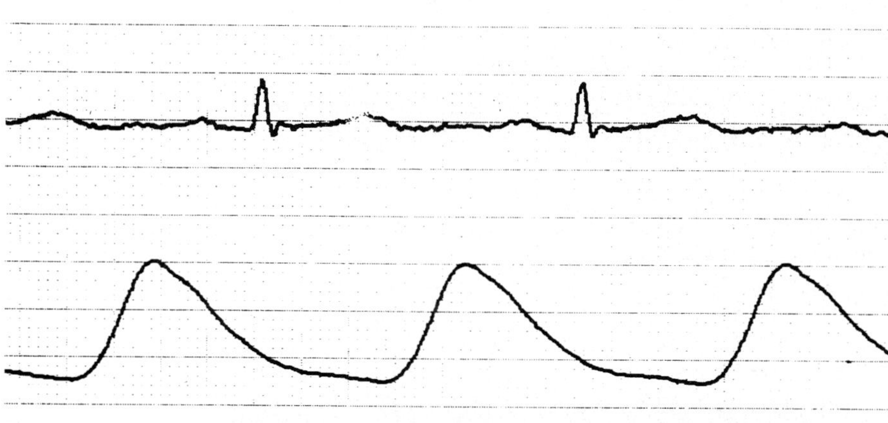

Fig. 4. Electrocardiogram (ECG) and arterial trace of in vivo test. Heart rate, 87 bpm; mean arterial pressure, 57 mmHg, systole/diastole, 87/21

In Vivo Test

During the assist period of the experiments, a preload of approximately 15 mmHg was maintained by the administration of intravenous lactated Ringer's solution. In the case of increased afterload, sodium nitroprusside was administered.

Left ventricular support was initiated in a 1:1 fashion and was changed to 1:2 only in those cases in which a significant increase in heart rate was observed. The VAD was able to maintain circulatory support and fully replace the animal's left ventricular function (Fig. 4). Urine output did not change during the experiments, and haematuria was not observed. During the last hour of the final two procedures, the left anterior descending coronary artery was ligated, resulting in acute severe ventricular dysfunction; however, the VAD successfully supported the circulation.

Discussion

In a limited, but significant number of patients, myocardial dysfunction develops with such severity that conventional treatment and intra-aortic balloon counterpulsation becomes ineffective. Profound cardiogenic shock develops and death ensues unless an aggressive mechanical intervention is applied. Treatment of cardiogenic shock with mechanical cardiac support has taken many different directions since the early attempts. Numerous devices have been designed to support the circulation, and the overall international clinical results demonstrate adequate survival rates [6]. However, all these devices are very expensive, which has limited their widespread application. Cardiogenic shock is a serious universal problem, and the need for simple, cost-efficient devices is growing day by day [7].

Our results support the hypothesis that less complex VAD can be designed and used in conjunction with existing resources, such as counterpulsation consoles, to act as drive modules. This approach not only significantly reduces the cost, but it can make this type of therapy applicable to a wider population of patients. However, despite our promising results, we believe that utilisation of conventional prosthetic mechanical valves makes the manufacture of artificial left ventricles expensive; we are therefore currently working on the design of a trileaflet polyurethane valve (Fig. 5).

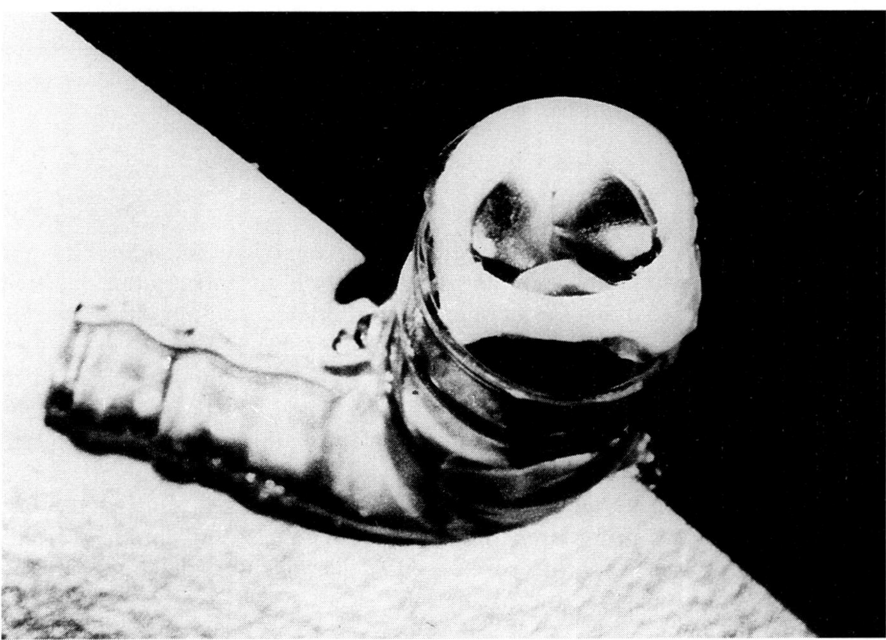

Fig. 5. Prototype of trileaflet polyurethane prosthetic valve

In conclusion, the data presented from this study demonstrates that VAD of simple design result in excellent haemodynamic performance in experimental animals when driven by conventional counterpulsation consoles. Further research is being conducted to evaluate performance for long-term support and to test clinical utility.

References

1. Baldwin TR, Slogoff S, Noon GP et al (1993) A model to predict survival at time of post-cardiotomy intraaortic balloon pump insertion. Ann Thorac Surg 55:908–913
2. Votapka TV, Pennington GD (1994) Circulatory assist devices in congestive heart failure. Cardiol Clin North Am 12:143–154
3. Minami K, El-Banayosi H, Posival H et al (1992) Improvement of survival rate in patients with cardiogenic shock by using nonpulsatile and pulsatile ventricular assist device. Int J Artif Org 15:715–721
4. Farrar DJ, Hill JD (1994) Recovery of major organ function in patients awaiting heart transplantation with Thoratec ventricular assist devices. J Heart Lung Transplant 13:1125–32
5. US Department of Health and Human Service (1992) Institutional Animal Care and Use Committee Guidebook. Public Health Services, National Institutes of Health, NIH Publ no 92–3415
6. Holman WL, Bourge CR, McGiffin DC, Kirklin JK (1994) Ventricular assist: experience with a pulsatile heterotopic device. Semin Thorac Cardiovasc Surg 3:147–153
7. Noriji C, Akutsu T, Koyanagi H, Kolff W (1992) Small soft left ventricular assist device powered by intraaortic balloon pump console for infants: a less expensive option. Artif Organs 16:382–385

Alterations in Serum Haptoglobin Concentration During the Early Phase of Myocardial Infarction

D. R. Bernard, M. R. Langlois, M. L. De Buyzere, and J. R. Delanghe

Introduction

Haptoglobin (Hp) is a haemoglobin-binding protein involved in the acute-phase reaction. Acute myocardial infarction (AMI) is characterised by inflammation and haemolysis. The aim of this study was to monitor the changes in Hp and free haemoglobin concentration during AMI as part of an investigation into the possible role of Hp in the pathogenesis of this disorder.

Methods

Hp and free haemoglobin were determined every 4 h using immunonephelometry techniques standardised according to methods recommended by the International Federation of Clinical Chemistry. Hp type was determined by starch gel electrophoresis of Hp-supplemented serum. AMI size was calculated using cumulative creatine kinase MB isoenzyme activity and myoglobin release. Acute-phase reaction upon admission was evaluated by measurement of C-reactive protein (CRP), a_1-anti-trypsin, a_1-acid glycoprotein and a_2-macroglobulin.

Results

Forty-five patients were investigated with the following Hp subtypes: Hp 1–1 ($n = 11$), Hp 2–1 ($n = 25$) and Hp 2–2 ($n = 9$). Reference and admission values for total Hp and subtypes together with the decease in concentration following AMI are shown in Table 1.

Following hospitalisation, the Hp concentration reached a minimal value at 9.6±5.8 h after admission, and the mean decrease corresponded to an average haemolysis of 10 ml red blood cells. The fall in Hp concentration was not related to infarct size (Spearman r, 0.17) nor to the type of treatment, but it was correlated with the initial Hp concentration (r, 0.78) and was more pronounced in men (0.53±0.57 g/l, $p < 0.05$) than in women (0.18±0.17 g/l). Of the acute-phase proteins that were measured on admission, only CRP was significantly increased ($p < 0.05$). In five patients with unstable angina, Hp concen-

Table 1. Reference and admission values for total haptoglobin (Hp) and subtypes and decrease in concentration after acute myocardial infarction (AMI)

	Total Hp	Hp subtype		
		Hp 1–1	Hp 2–1	Hp 2–2
Reference range (g/l)	0.97±0.46	1.24±0.51	0.99±0.41	0.76±0.42
Admission values (g/l)	1.95±0.94*	1.84±0.64*	1.98±0.79*	1.98±1.58*
Decrease after AMI (g/l)	–	0.30±0.19	0.52±0.24	0.56±0.65

Values are given as mean±SD.
* Significantly different from reference range values, $p<0.001$.

tration was normal upon hospital admission and showed no decrease during early hospitalisation.

Conclusions

Our study has shown that early AMI is preceded by a raised Hp and CRP concentration. After admission, the Hp concentration decreases and then rises as part of the acute-phase reaction. These changes, which are more pronounced in men, suggest a haemolytic process and may have a role in the pathogenesis of coronary occlusion and AMI.

References

1. Chapelle JP, Albert A, Smeets J et al (1982) Effect of the haptoglobin phenotype on the size of a myocardial infarct. N Eng J Med 307:457–463

Association of Interleukin-2 Receptor with Acute Myocardial Infarction

L. Xuguo, X. Yuzhong, Z. Shilin, and Y. Lijun

Introduction

Acute myocardial infarction (AMI) is one of the leading causes of death in China. The aim of this study was to determine the possible involvement of cytokines in AMI by measurement of soluble interleukin-2 receptor (IL-2R) in patients with AMI or angina pectoris (AP).

Methods

The subjects in this study were 20 patients with AMI, 20 patients with AP and 20 normal subjects as controls. Parameters measured included IL-2R by sandwich enzyme-linked immunosorbent assay (ELISA), circulating immuno-complex (CIC) and serum immunoglobulins IgM, IgG and IgA.

Results

Results from the measurements in the three groups are shown in Table 1. The IL-2R and CIC levels in the two patient groups were significantly higher than in the controls; IgG was significantly higher in the two patient groups, while IgM was significantly lower.

Table 1. Measurements of interleukin-2 receptor (IL-2R), circulating immunocomplex (CIC) and serum immunoglobulins in patients with acute myocardial infarction (AMI) or angina pectoris (AP)

	IL-2R (U/ml)	CIC (μg/ml)	IgA (μg/ml)	IgG (μg/ml)	IgM (μg/ml)
Controls ($n = 20$)	294±65	0.17±0.08	2279±1550	10188±4510	1576±694
AP ($n = 20$)	432±55[**]	0.32±0.08[**]	2038±777	13647±5118[*]	936±75[**]
AMI ($n = 20$)	389±58[*]	0.46±0.09[**]	2493±1056	14515±5165[*]	948±479[**]

Values are expressed as mean±SD.

* $p < 0.05$; ** $p < 0.01$.

Conclusions

These results suggest that human lymphocytes are activated in vivo in patients with cardiovascular disease and that IL-2R levels may be a useful biochemical indicator of disease activity.

Changes in Expression of Interleukin-2 Receptor and Interleukin-2 Production on Peripheral Blood Mononuclear Cells in Cardiac Surgery Patients

L. Ai-lin, T. Yu-ke, and J. Shi-ao

Introduction

Many patients who undergo cardiac bypass surgery develop postsurgical complications, including infectious disease and multiple organ failure. It has been hypothesised that these complications may arise from disturbances to the immune system caused by events which take place during cardiac surgery, such as prolonged anaesthesia, the bypass process itself or cardiac surgical procedures. This study was aimed at evaluating the changes in cell-mediated immunity which take place during and after bypass surgery.

Methods

Measurements were carried out on blood from 40 patients undergoing cardiac bypass surgery. Thirty patients undergoing cholecystectomy or subtotal gastrectomy were selected as the control group. Blood samples were taken from the patients prior to anaesthesia, 55 min after anaesthesia was induced, at the end of cardiopulmonary bypass and at 1, 7 and 14 days postoperatively. Peripheral blood mononuclear cells (PBMC) were separated by a gradient density technique. Expression rates of interleukin-2 receptor (IL-2R) were detected with indirect immunofluorescence using a anti-Tac monoclonal antibody. In vitro IL-2 synthesis was carried out by stimulation of phytohaemagglutinin.

Results

Pre-, peri- and postoperative results are shown in Table 1.

Conclusions

The patients undergoing cardiac surgery showed significant falls in IL-2R expression and IL-2 production after inducement of anaesthesia, and this re-

Table 1. Pre-, peri- and postoperative expression of interleukin (IL)-2 receptor (IL-2R) and production of IL-2

	IL-2R expression (U/ml)		IL-2 production (ng/l)	
	Cardiac	Control	Cardiac	Control
Pre-anaesthetic	48.81±10.98	54.40±5.23	99.08±26.78	91.29±15.15
55 min post-anaesthetic	39.14±11.77**	52.27±4.32	63.58±10.68***	90.52±9.27
End of bypass	37.00±11.61**	55.29±5.31	61.45±5.0***	89.91±6.71
Postoperative day 1	36.00±11.17***	54.44±6.19	54.75±6.36***	88.19±7.80
Postoperative day 7	39.67±10.36*	56.27±7.50	60.50±6.80***	86.62±9.20
Postoperative day 14	47.00±9.02	55.27±8.27	70.00±8.42***	87.19±9.17

Results are expressed as mean±SD.

* $p<0.005$ (comparison with pre-anaesthetic values); ** $p<0.01$ (comparison with pre-anaesthetic values); *** $p<0.001$ (comparison with pre-anaesthetic values).

duction was maintained in the postoperative period. These decreases, which were not exhibited by the patients undergoing general surgery, correlated with a much higher rate of postoperative infection in the cardiac patients, and it is believed that this may be due to the alterations in cytokine expression and production.

Interrelationship Between Serum and Cerebrospinal Fluid Enzymes in Comatose Patients

P. Martens, A. Mullie, and M. Bourgeois

Introduction

In patients who are comatose following a cardiac arrest, it has been recommended that the measurement of creatine kinase BB isoenzyme CK-BB, aspartate aminotransferase (AST) and lactic dehydrogenase (LDH) in cerebrospinal fluid (CSF) collected 48 h after the arrest can assist in the decision of whether to continue therapy. Recently, measurement of serum neurone-specific enolase (NSE) 24 h after arrest has also been advocated for the same purpose. The aim of this study was to compare the prognostic value of serum NSE with CSF enzyme levels in diagnosing reversible brain injury.

Methods

The subjects of this study were 16 patients who had suffered a cardiac arrest but were now comatose. In addition to collection of serum samples for NSE measurement, all patients underwent a lumbar puncture and CK-BB, AST and LDH were measured in the CSF. γ-Subunits of NSE were measured in serum by a standardised polyclonal radioimmunoassay supplied by Pharmacia (Uppsala, Sweden). The relationship between serum NSE and each of the CSF enzymes was tested using the Spearman's correlation coefficient. The outcome in each patient was either 0 (corresponding to CNS failure; cerebral performance category, CPC, 5) or 1 (corresponding to awake; CPC, 1–3).

Results

The individual patient results are shown in Table 1. Serum NSE correlated significantly with CSF CK-BB, but not with the other enzymes. In three patients who had a poor outcome, either serum NSE or CSF-BB were unexpectedly lower than the threshold value and falsely indicative of a favourable outcome (patient nos. 8, 9 and 12), while in one patient (no. 13) both activities were lower than the threshold value.

Table 1. Serum neurone-specific enolase (S-NSE), CK-BB, aspartate aminotransferase (AST) and lactic dehydrogenase (LDH) levels in comatose patients

Patients	S-NSE (ng/ml)	CK-BB (U/l)	AST (U/l)	LDH (U/l)	Outcome[a]
1	15.1	4	33	54	1+cardiac failure
2	10.7	8	23	32	1
3	22.0	44	414	427	0
4	36.8	1	NA	23	1
5	158	219	147	127	0
6	50.5	273	148	121	0
7	65	26	424	623	0
8	25.9	17	387	478	0
9	15.6	26	NA	57	0
10	49.2	126	38	38	0
11	45.5	156	NA	361	0
12	19.0	18	69	92	0
13	11.5	3	NA	44	0
14	46.0	85	1206	1488	0
15	24.0	1192	996	1115	0
16	15.2	1	16	13	?+cardiac failure
r	0.64	$p<0.01$	0.53 (NS)	0.48 (NS)	
Threshold	18	20	62	82	

NS, not significant.

[a] 0, CNS failure; 1, awake.

Conclusions

Measurement of serum NSE at 24 h after cardiac arrest is a cheap test that is easy to perform for the early assessment of hypoxic/ischaemic encephalo-pathy after cardiac arrest.

Role of Transoesophageal Echocardiography in Patients with Severe Blunt Chest Trauma for the Diagnosis and Management of Traumatic Disruption of the Aorta

P. Vignon and P. Lagrange

Introduction

Traumatic disruption of the aorta (TDA) is a life-threatening injury which requires rapid surgery. Although aortography is considered the gold standard for the diagnosis of TDA, transoesophageal echocardiography (TEE) has recently emerged as an alternative diagnostic technique. We conducted a prospective study to (a) describe the TEE signs associated with TDA and their potential impact on patient management, (b) evaluate the accuracy of TEE for the diagnosis of TDA and (c) evaluate the value of routine TEE to rule out TDA in trauma patients presenting with a non-enlarged mediastinum on chest X-ray.

Methods

Over a 2 year period, victims of violent deceleration accidents underwent both a TEE examination and a 100 cm anteroposterior chest X-ray on admission. Aortography was obtained when (a) TEE indicated a diagnosis of TDA, (b) the mediastinum was widened (>8 cm) on presentation chest X-ray, or (c) TEE was not diagnostic. TEE findings associated with TDA were compared with those encountered in patients sustaining an acute aortic dissection (AAD) during the same period. All TEE diagnoses of TDA were corroborated by surgery or necropsy.

Results

Of 80 patients enrolled in the study, 72 had suffered trauma (mean age, 38±16 years), while 18 had confirmed AAD (mean age, 57±15 years). TEE indicated a diagnosis of subadventitial TDA in 11 patients (rapid surgery), allowing the description of echocardiographic differential diagnostic criteria to distinguish TDA from AAD. TEE also indicated a diagnosis of traumatic intimal tear in three patients (successful conservative management with TEE follow-up). When compared with aortography in 32 patients with a widened mediastinum, TEE had a sensitivity and specificity for the diagnosis of TDA of 91% and 100%, respectively, while two thirds of intimal tears were not noted on angiograms. Among 40 patients with non-enlarged mediastinum, TEE indicated a diagnosis of TDA in two patients. The frequency of chest X-ray findings commonly used as indicators to perform aortography was similar in patients with ($n=6$) and without ($n=34$) mediastinal haematoma during TEE examination.

Conclusions

TEE allows differentiation between TDA and AAD and yields useful information for the management of traumatic aortic injuries. In experienced hands, TEE is an accurate, non-invasive imaging modality for the diagnosis of TDA, and its routine use in victims of violent deceleration accidents, even with normal mediastinum on presentation chest X-ray, may decrease the number of undiagnosed TDA.

Haemodynamic Effects of Different Modes of Positive-Pressure Mechanical Ventilation

T. Samir, A.A. El-Fattah, and S. Mokhtar

Introduction

Many critically ill patients require mechanical ventilation, which directly affects cardiovascular performance by changing lung volume or intrathoracic pressure. Furthermore, oxygen delivery (DO_2) to the various organs is a product of regional blood flow and oxygen content. The aim of this study was to compare the effects of different modes of positive-pressure ventilation on circulatory dynamics and oxygen transport.

Methods

The subjects of this study were 20 patients admitted to the intensive care unit over a period of 5 months; there were nine males and 11 females, with a mean age of 50.1 ± 15 years. Each patient was subject to bedside Swan-Ganz catheterisation, central venous and arterial line insertion and calculation of cardiac output (CO) by thermodilution. The following other haemodynamic and biochemical parameters were measured: heart rate (HR), arterial blood pressure (ABP), central venous pressure (CVP), pulmonary artery pressure (PAP), pulmonary capillary wedge pressure (PCWP), cardiac index (CI), systemic vascular resistance (SVR), pulmonary vascular resistance, DO_2, and arterial blood gas analysis. These haemodynamic variables were obtained during a control period of continuous mandatory ventilation (CMV) mode, then CMV plus positive end-expiratory pressure (PEEP), synchronised intermittent mandatory ventilation (SIMV), SIMV plus PEEP, continuous positive airway pressure (CPAP) and pressure support ventilation (PSV), with 30 min intermission on control CMV prior to institution of each mode.

Results

The results for the haemodynamic variables obtained with the various ventilatory modes were compared to those obtained with CMV and are shown in Table 1.

Table 1. Effect of different modes of positive-pressure mechanical ventilation on haemodynamic and biochemical parameters

Parameter	Mode/variable					
	CMV	CMV+PEEP	SIMV	SIMV+PEEP	CPAP	PSV
HR (min)	112	113	112	115	119**	117*
ABP (mmHg)	86.6	84.2	87.7	81	83	81*
CVP (mmHg)	8.7	11**	8.7	10*	11.5**	12.4**
PAP (mmHg)	26.9	27.9*	24.5**	25.5**	27.4	28.2
PCWP (mmHg)	15.4	17.1*	13.1*	17.7	15.7	17.3*
CO (l/min)	6.6	5.8**	6.9*	6.2	6.1	5.8**
CI (l/min/m^2)	3.6	3.2**	3.8	3.5	3.4*	3.2**
SVR (dyne/s/cm^5)	931.5	1007	884.5	128	567	112.5
PVR (dyne/s/cm^5)	140	146	951	117**	517	119.2
DO$_2$ (ml/min)	518	476	946.5	138.5	509	108.9
PaO$_2$ (mmHg)	115.8	120.1	960	149	481	120.6

Results expressed as mean changes from baseline continuous mandatory ventilation (CMV) mode values.

HR, heart rate; ABP, arterial blood pressure; CVP, central venous pressure; PAP, pulmonary artery pressure; PCWP, pulmonary capillary wedge pressure; CO, cardiac output; CI, cardiac index; SVR, systemic vascular resistance; PVR, pulmonary vascular resistance; DO$_2$, oxygen delivery; PEEP, positive end-expiratory pressure; SIMV, synchronised intermittent mandatory ventilation; CPAP, continuous positive airway pressure; PSV, pressure support ventilation. *$p<0.05$; **$p<0.01$.

Compared to the haemodynamic parameters of the CMV mode, SIMV showed the highest DO$_2$ (9.4%), with significant improvement of the CO (4.5%), PAP (9%) and PCWP (15%) and little effect on SVR (5%) and PVR (8.5%). Both the addition of PEEP to CMV and, surprisingly, PSV, which is often used for weaning, had worse effects on haemodynamics, with reductions in DO$_2$ (8% and 7%, respectively), CO (12% and 12%, respectively), ABP (2.7% and 6%, respectively) and increases in PAP (3.7% and 5%, respectively), PCWP (11% and 12%, respectively), SVR (8% and 3%, respectively) and PVR (4.3% and 6.5%, respectively). Other modes of CMV, CPAP and SIMV plus PEEP had insignificant effects on circulatory dynamics, PaO$_2$ and ultimately DO$_2$.

Conclusions

We conclude from this study that positive-pressure ventilation has adverse effects on circulatory dynamics. The choice of ventilation mode and the best weaning policy should therefore be guided by the underlying clinical condition and followed up haemodynamically by non-invasive and, if necessary, invasive means.

Coronary Reserve and Myocardial Metabolism in Patients with Angina and Normal Coronary Arteriogram

A. El-Sherif, S. A. El-Shafee, A. Zaki, R. Bahgat, and M. S. Mokhtar

Introduction

Not all cardiac patients with angina have abnormal coronary angiograms. The aim of this study was to evaluate the coronary reserve by other tests, including coronary pacing and studies of myocardial metabolism (MM).

Methods

Coronary flow reserve (CFR) and MM were assessed in 16 patients, four males and 12 females (mean age, 43.4 years). Three of the patients were diabetic, four had hypertension and three had abnormal lipid profiles. Similar studies were carried out in five control subjects. All patients had clinical evidence of ischaemia with a positive treadmill test and/or positive thallium scan, but all had patent epicardial coronary arteries. All patients underwent the insertion of a flow-directed Swan-Ganz catheter, a coronary sinus catheter and an arterial line. Haemodynamic measurements included arterial blood pressure, cardiac output (CO), pulmonary artery pressure (PAP), pulmonary capillary wedge pressure (PCWP), systemic (SVR) and pulmonary vascular resistance (PVR), coronary sinus flow (CSF), coronary resistance (CR) and cardiac indices. Biochemical parameters were measured in arterial and coronary sinus blood and included the following parameters: pH and blood gases, lactate, pyruvate, sodium, potassium and glucose. Both haemodynamic and biochemical parameters were measured at rest and at maximal coronary dilation achieved by incremental coronary sinus pacing and by dipyridamole (0.56 mg/kg).

Results

Table 1 compares the resting haemodynamic and biochemical measurements in the 12 patients with the values obtained after pacing and dipyrimadole treatment.

Table 1. Resting haemodynamic and biochemical measurements and results after pacing and dipyrimadole treatment

	CSF (ml/min)		Lactate(mmol/l)			PCWP (mmHg)	
	CSF	(% change)	Arter.	CS	Consumption	(PCWP)	(% change)
Resting	124		2.6	2.1	−20	9	
Pacing	136	+9.6	2.8	2.9	+3	18	+100
Dipyridamole	141	+14	2.7	2.9	+8	11	+22

CSF, coronary sinus flow; PCWP, pulmonary capillary wedge pressure.

Cardiac output in the patients increased 0% and 13% with pacing and with dipyridamole compared to the control subjects, in which it increased 40% and 50%, respectively. The patients also showed a much lower increase in CSF than the controls (9.6% and 14% compared to 80% and 90% with pacing and dipyridamole, respectively), and extraction of lactate in the patients was 3% and 8% with pacing and dipyridamole, respectively, compared to 40% and 45% in the controls.

Conclusions

Of the 16 patients, 12 had reduced lactate extraction associated with other haemodynamic and electrocardiographic evidence of myocardial ischaemia. We conclude that patients with angina but apparently normal coronary arteries exhibit impaired CSF and MM manifested by reduced lactate extraction. These abnormalities could only be revealed by CSF measurement.

Early Detection of Successful Coronary Reperfusion Based on Serum Levels of Human Heart-Type Cytoplasmic Fatty Acid-Binding Protein

J. Ishii, Y. Nagamura, N. Masanori, Y. Watanabe, H. Hishida, T. Tanaka, and K. Karamura

Introduction

Heart-type cytoplasmic fatty acid-binding protein (H-FABPc) is a cytoplasmic low molecular weight protein similar to myoglobin. The skeletal myoglobin content is approximately twice that of the heart, while the concentration of H-FABPc in striated muscle is only 10%–50% of that in cardiac muscle. The aim of this study was to assess the usefulness of H-FABPc measurement in the early detection of successful coronary reperfusion.

Methods

We measured H-FABPc and myoglobin in 45 patients undergoing percutaneous transluminal coronary reperfusion (by urokinase or tissue-type plasminogen activator) or angioplasty within 6 h after acute myocardial infarction. Coronary angiography was performed every 5 min during reperfusion therapy to identify the onset of reperfusion. In 30 patients with reperfusion (23 patients with Thrombolysis in Myocardial Infaction trial grade 3, and seven patients with grade 2), blood samples were obtained before reperfusion and 15, 30 and 60 min after reperfusion. In 15 patients without reperfusion, samples were obtained just before initiation of treatment and 15, 30 and 60 min after treatment. H-FABPc was measured by competitive enzyme immunoassay, and myoglobin by turbidometric latex agglutination method.

Results

The concentration of H-FABPc or myoglobin at each time interval was expressed as a ratio of the concentration before reperfusion or treatment (H-FABPc after/H-FABPc before). The H-FABPc ratio increased sharply after the onset of reperfusion, peaking at 41 ± 18 min, and decreased rapidly thereafter. The predictive accuracy of the two markers for reperfusion is shown in Table 1.

Table 1. Predictive acccuracy of the concentration of heart-type cytoplasmic fatty acid-binding protein (H-FABPc) and myoglobin

Time after reperfusion (min) >2.4[b]	Predictive accuracy (%)	
	H-FABPc ratio >1.8[a]	Myoglobin ratio
15	93	93
30	98	96
60	100	100

[a] Mean±2SD at 60 min in 15 patients without reperfusion.
[b] Published criteria [1].

Conclusions

H-FABPc and myoglobin ratios detected successful reperfusion as early as 15 min after the onset of reperfusion and were highly accurate in detecting reperfusion within 60 min of the onset of treatment. The predictive accuracy of the H-FABPc ratio was similar to that of the myoglobin ratio.

References

1. Ishii J, Nomura M, Ando T et al (1994) Early detection of successful coronary reperfusion based on serum myoglobin concentration: comparison with serum creatine kinase isoenzyme MB activity. Am J Heart J 128:641–648

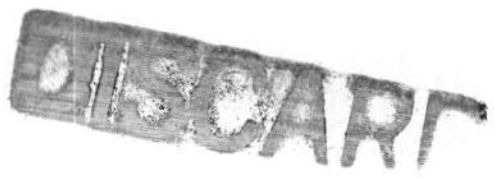

Cardiac Troponin I as a Marker for Perioperative Myocardial Ischaemia in Non-cardiac Surgery Patients

B. W. Bottiger, J. Motsch, P. Teschendorf, G. Rehmert, R. Gust, M. Zorn, M. Schweizer, and E. Martin

Introduction

Episodes of perioperative myocardial ischaemia (PMI) occur in 18%–74% of non-cardiac surgery patients with coronary artery disease (CAD) [1]. Patients with PMI have a higher risk of suffering adverse cardiac outcome postoperatively. Early diagnosis and treatment of PMI may improve outcome in these patients. Cardiac troponin I is a new marker for myocardial cell damage, and the aim of this study was to investigate its diagnostic value in detecting PMI.

Methods

The subjects of this study were 55 patients (mean age, 65±9 years) who were undergoing vascular surgery. The patients either had documented CAD or at least two of the following risk factors: age >65 years, smoker, diabetes mellitus, hypertension, hypercholesterolaemia >240 mg/dl. Twelve-lead electrocardiogram (ECG) recordings were carried out preoperatively, immediately after the operation and at 20, 48, 72 and 84 h postoperatively. They were analysed by an independent cardiologist for signs of PMI (new ST segment depression >0.2 mV and/or new T inversion). Blood samples were taken preoperatively, immediately after the operation and at 4, 8, 12, 16, 20, 24, 32, 40, 48, 60, 72 and 84 h postoperatively for measurement of cardiac troponin I using the Baxter Stratus method (Baxter Diagnostics, Miami, FL).

Results

In 44% of patients, PMI was documented on ECG. Table 1 shows a comparison of cardiac troponin I (cut-off value, 1.6 ng/ml) and ECG results. Sensitivity, specificity and predictive values of cardiac troponin I versus ECG are shown in Table 2.

Table 1. Comparison of cardiac troponin I and electrocardiogram (ECG) results

Cardiac troponin I level	Patients (n)	
	PMI[a]	No PMI[a]
>1.6 ng/ml	19	2
≤1.6 ng/ml	5	29

PMI, peri-operative myocardial ischaemia.
[a] 12-lead ECG.

Table 2. Sensitivity, specificity and predictive values of cardiac troponin I versus 12-lead electrocardiogram (ECG)

	Cardiac troponin I vs. 12-lead ECG
Sensitivity (%)	79
Specificity (%)	94
Positive predictive value (%)	91
Negative predictive value (%)	85

Conclusions

These results demonstrate that troponin I is a highly sensitive and specific marker for ECG-documented PMI in patients with or at risk of CAD. Thus measurement of cardiac troponin I may be useful for the identification of CAD patients who have to undergo non-cardiac surgery and are at risk of an adverse postoperative cardiac outcome.

References

1. Mangano DT (1990) Perioperative cardiac morbidity. Anaesthesiology 72:153–184

Endogenous Nitric Oxide and the Low Systemic Vascular Resistance Syndrome Following Cardiac Surgery

P. S. Myles, C. Leong, and J. Curry

Introduction

The low systemic vascular resistance (SVR) syndrome following cardiac surgery and cardiopulmonary bypass (CPB) increases patient risk and time spent in the intensive care unit [1] and involves up to 1500 cardiac surgical patients each year throughout Australia. Because septic shock and the low SVR syndrome have similar adverse haemodynamic effects, it is possible that similar mechanisms may be operating in both abnormalities. Septic shock may result in excessive production of the endogenous vasodilator nitric oxide (NO), which is eventually metabolised to nitrate and nitrite [2, 3]. The aim of this study was to test the hypothesis that intrinsic NO production is elevated in patients with low SVR syndrome.

Methods

Subjects with low SVR were recruited together with control subjects with normal SVR and were matched for age, sex and surgery. Blood and urine samples were taken in the intensive care unit 4–24 h after surgery. Nitrate levels were measured by gas chromatography mass spectrometry [3]. Statistical analysis was done using the Wilcoxon signed rank test, Spearman rank correlation and logistic regression.

Results

A total of 44 subjects were recruited, and the results of various parameters in the patient and control groups is shown in Table 1.

Low SVR patients had a higher cardiac output ($p < 0.001$), required longer ventilation ($p = 0.02$) and spent longer in the intensive care unit ($p = 0.02$). There was no difference in the serum or urine nitrates, nor in other predictors of low SVR. There was a negative association between CPB temperature and nitrate level (r, –0.36).

Table 1. Comparison of parameters in patients with low systemic vacular resistance (SVR) syndrome and controls

Parameter	Patients ($n=15$)		Controls ($n=29$)	
	Median	Range	Median	Range
CO (l/min)	6.63	3.7–11.8	4.37	4.08–5.75
SVR (dyne/s/cm^5)	676	459–840	1297	1049–1875
Serum NO (µmol/l)	58	39–77	62	34–85
Urine NO (µmol/l)	399	158–992	404	193–1212
Extubation (h)	17.8	4.9–45.3	8.7	0.9–800
Discharge from ICU (days)	2.5	0.8–42	1.2	0.6–33

CO, cardiac output; ICU, intensive care unit.

Conclusions

This study found no evidence of endogenous NO production as a cause of the low SVR syndrome following cardiac surgery. It confirms the poor outcome in this group, including the cost implications of prolonged mechanical ventilation and longer stay in the intensive care unit and supports the need for further research into this disorder.

References

1. Myles PS, Olenikov I, Bujor MA et al (1993) ACE-inhibitors, calcium antagonists and low systemic vascular resistance following cardiopulmonary bypass. A case-control study. Med J Aust 158:675–677
2. Evans T, Carpenter A, Kinderman H et al (1993) Evidence of increased nitric oxide production in patients with the sepsis syndrome. Circ Shock 41:77–81
3. Winlaw DS, Smythe GA, Keogh AM et al (1994) Increased nitric oxide production in heart failure. Lancet 344:373–374

Blood Gases – Electrolytes – Trace Elements

Towards Clinically Useful Expert Systems in Critical Care: Locally Managed Interpretation of Arterial Blood Gas Data

G. A. Edwards, P. J. Compton, P. J. Preston, and B. Ho Kang

Abstract

Clinical pathology tests generate large volumes of data for critical care clinicians, and "data overload" can impede clinical decision making. Bedside arterial blood gas (ABG) analysis is compounding this problem. Expert systems (ES) have great potential to support clinicians' work, but few ES are in routine use. The complexity of knowledge acquisition (KA) leads to poor productivity in the development phase and requires specialist knowledge engineering (KE) skills. This has been termed the knowledge acquisition "bottleneck". We have devised a novel algorithm, ripple-down rules (RDR), that essentially eliminates the KE bottleneck. The Pathology Expert Interpretative Reporting System (PEIRS), an RDR ES, interprets a broad range of pathology reports (including thyroid function tests, ABG, cardiac enzymes and a range of hormone assays) and has been in routine use for over 4 years. With over 2100 rules, PEIRS is one of the few large medical ES in routine use, and apparently the only large ES built entirely by a pathologist without specialist KE skills or support. A key finding from PEIRS was that its simple KA strategy enabled localisation of its knowledge, e.g. local protocols for interpretation and management. This localisation was essential for gaining the acceptance of the system by the pathologists.

While PEIRS successfully automated the interpretation of ABG reports, extension to bedside decision support was limited by its restriction of a single interpretative comment per report. A new algorithm, multiple-classification RDR (MC-RDR), addresses this issue. We compared conventional RDR and MC-RDR by building prototype ES for ABG interpretation. Data included pH, PCO_2, PO_2, calculated bicarbonate, base excess and patient's age on up to five sequential specimens. Interpretations such as "resolving respiratory acidosis, metabolic compensation" were based on local criteria, e.g. "severe hypoxaemia" if PO_2 is less than 59 mmHg. After 262 cases, MC-RDR was far more compact than RDR (262 vs. 442 total rule conditions), simpler to maintain (109 vs. 184 rules; 22 vs. 129 comments) and matured earlier (84% vs. 30% accuracy for the last 50 cases). The KA task for the local expert was marginally more complex with MC-RDR, but this was more than offset by the substantial overall reduction in KA requirements.

We have shown that MC-RDR is more compact than RDR, and KA is far more efficient. Its rapid maturation supports application in routine clinical care and would suit an embedded decision support system for an ABG analyser. By enabling localisation, we believe that MC-RDR redefines the role of medical ES and that real-time MC-RDR ES will soon be helping critical care clinicians reduce data overload in their daily practice.

Introduction

Critical care medicine is a data-rich environment. Clinicians need to assimilate large volumes of data from a range of sources, including physiological monitors and laboratory tests, when formulating rapid patient management decisions. The recent trend of installing biochemical analysers, such as blood gas and oximetry instruments, in critical care units is increasing the amount of raw data generated at the bedside.

There is ample evidence that data overload hinders decision making, in medicine as in other areas of human endeavour, such as aviation [1]. Critical care clinicians are already exposed to electronic signal interpretation systems that generate alarms. However, these instruments are of limited value, as they tend to generate many distracting false-positive alarms. As Coiera [2] observed, technology companies spend millions of dollars developing sophisticated alarms that clinical staff ignore. As a consequence, considerable efforts are underway to build intelligent clinical decision support systems that can assist the doctor in managing clinical data [3, 4]. There is already evidence that computerised interpretation, including clinical alerts and biochemical diagnosis, can improve patient outcomes, compliance with management protocols and medical education [5–7].

Clinical Decision Support for Arterial Blood Gas Data

Bedside ABG analysis has been made possible by the development of compact, robust and reliable analysers. While continuous in vivo monitoring of ABG holds some promise, it seems likely that, for the foreseeable future, most ABG will be performed in vitro, by medical or other clinical staff, in discrete episodes [8]. ABG data is generally accessed directly from the instrument. In the future, data may also be accessed from bedside clinical workstations that display a variety of patient data. As patient management decisions based on ABG data tend to be made immediately, a decision support system needs to be embedded either in the analyser itself or in the bedside electronic patient record.

A number of artificial intelligence approaches have been used for interpretation of ABG [9–11]. However, none of these have reached routine use. Indeed, very few interpretative systems have found application in any routine medical setting. One of the prime obstacles to the transfer of artificial intelligence technology to the bedside is the complexity of KA. KA traditionally relies on close cooperation between a domain expert, e.g. a pathologist, and a computer scientist with specialist skills in KE. This is a complex and tedious process, with the result that productivity in development is poor, and the life span of production systems is limited. Indeed, most systems do not reach routine operation for this reason. This KE bottleneck is a major focus of artificial intelligence research [12].

Ripple-Down Rules

ES are computer programmes that classify data using "if–then" rules. The advantage of this approach is that the rules are generally in a form that can be comprehended by humans (such as "if: WINGS then: BIRD"). While experts can readily provide simple rules for interpretation, different contexts requiring modifications to rules are soon encountered (such as "if: LEGS=6 then: INSECT; if: FIXED WINGS then: AEROPLANE). Both the rules and the inferencing process (which determines the manner in which the rules are evaluated) become highly complex. The KE bottleneck is quickly reached and, as for other artificial intelligence approaches, few ES have seen routine operation in medicine.

Recently, we have described a novel ES strategy, RDR, that largely eliminates the KE bottleneck. RDR allows domain experts to maintain their own knowledge bases independently, without KE skills or support [13]. We have validated the RDR approach in PEIRS, an ES for interpreting chemical pathology reports [14]. PEIRS has been in routine operation for over 4 years. As one of the few medical expert systems in routine operation, PEIRS is unique in that its knowledge base has been built and maintained entirely by a professional pathologist as part of his routine duties. PEIRS currently contains over 2100 rules and interprets test results for a broad range of pathology tests, including thyroid function tests, ABG, catecholamines, cardiac enzymes, glucose tolerance tests and a range of hormone levels.

Localisation and the Evolving Knowledge Base

One of the major findings from PEIRS was the notion that ES in medicine can never be considered complete. Medical knowledge, and its application in health care environments, is constantly evolving. Evolving knowledge and practice need to be incorporated into ES if they are to remain current and relevant. In addition, there was considerable local knowledge inherent in many of PEIRS interpretations, such as local protocols for interpretation and follow-up testing as well as locally derived reference intervals and areas of special expertise. Indeed, the pathologists were only satisfied with PEIRS' performance if its interpretations adequately reflected their local expertise. Clinicians in critical care will also demand that an ABG ES is consistent with their knowledge, practice and beliefs. Clancey [15] has recently emphasised the primacy of local context for interpretative strategies that are acceptable to clinicians. This is especially relevant when doctors seek to apply established care guidelines to individual patients: "good practice involves knowing when to violate a rule, when a new classification might be appropriate, when an alternative interpretation of a guideline might better fit the values of medicine."

This notion of the locally evolving knowledge base challenges conventional approaches to ES development, where the emphasis has been on pre-implementation accuracy for essentially static systems. The ease of knowledge base maintenance in PEIRS enabled it to adapt readily to change. Similarly, decision support systems for ABG in critical care must support modification by local experts. This process must be fast and simple and not interfere with routine patient care activities. It must also evolve sufficiently rapidly so that its output remains current.

"Multiple Classification" Problem

While PEIRS successfully automated the interpretation of ABG reports, comprehensive interpretation was limited by the restriction (inherent in RDR) to a single interpretative comment. ABG data commonly contain multiple clinically important states. PEIRS was only able to deal with this situation (the "multiple classification" problem) by combining all disorders into a single comment. This leads to a serious problem of combinatorial explosion. PEIRS contains hundreds of ABG rules, and additional rules are still required. Subsequently, we have developed a new algorithm, MC-RDR, to address this issue [16]. Theoretical studies suggest that MC-RDR produces compact knowledge bases [17], but it has yet to be tested in a true multiple-classification domain. In addition, the impact of MC-RDR on the expert's ability to manage the system unaided has not been determined.

We therefore sought to investigate the utility of MC-RDR for interpreting ABG data. Of particular importance is the ability of MC-RDR to solve the multiple-classification problem and the extent to which ongoing management of an evolving knowledge base can be sustained by local experts in critical care.

Aims

The aims of this study were to investigate the utility of MC-RDR for building ES for interpreting ABG data for critical care units and to define the implications of MC-RDR for local expert management of an evolving medical knowledge base.

Materials and Methods

Ripple-Down Rules and Multiple-Classification Ripple-Down Rules

The inferencing algorithms and KA methodologies for conventional RDR and MC-RDR have been described in detail elsewhere [13, 16]. However, a brief description of the key features of RDR and their modification for MC-RDR is provided here for explanation.

Ripple-Down Rules

An RDR ES is a binary decision tree. Each node has rule conditions ("if" statements) and a conclusion ("then" statement). If a case satisfies a node, its "true" branch is evaluated. Otherwise, the "false" branch is evaluated. The final conclusion for a case is that of the last satisfied node.

Consider the simple RDR tree shown in Fig. 1. Any case with "wings" and "legs = 6" will be classified as "insect". Note that node 2 is only evaluated if node 1 is true.

Next, consider a case we wish to classify as "bee": wings = true, legs = 6, sting = true, social = true, striped=true. This case currently will be classified as "insect". To reclassify it, we need a new rule.

Nodes are never deleted or modified. New nodes are attached at the end of the node sequence that has generated the incorrect conclusion. In addition, only valid rules are allowed. This is achieved by storing the case ("cornerstone case") that prompted the addition of a rule. A valid rule is one that will correctly interpret the new case, but will not be satisfied by the pre-

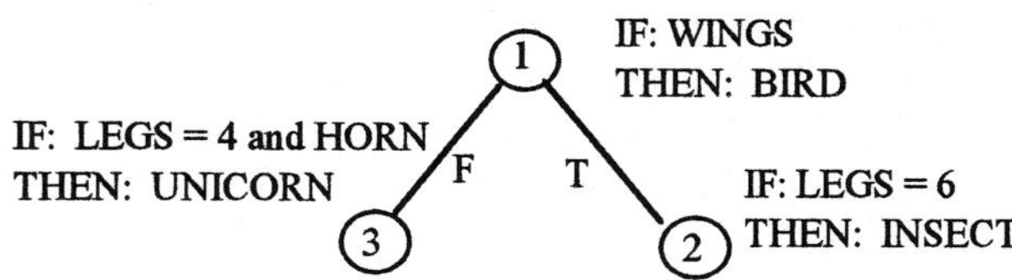

Fig. 1. A simple ripple-down rule tree (RDR)

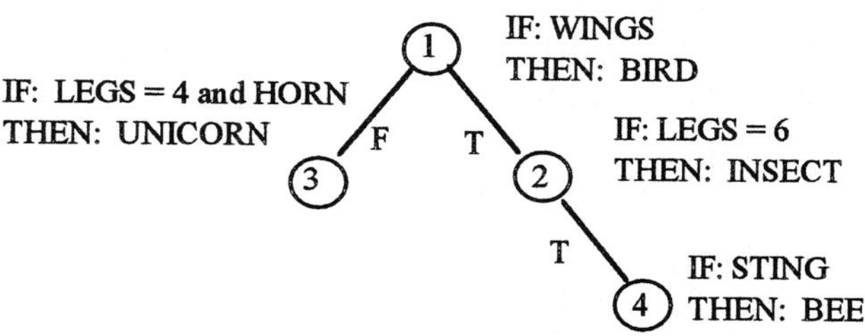

Fig. 2. A new rule added

vious cornerstone case. When adding a rule, we choose conditions from a list of *differences* between the current case and the previous cornerstone case.

To reclassify the above case as "bee", we examine the cornerstone case for rule 2: wings = true, legs = 6, sting = false, colour = black, striped = true. The system will generate the following difference list: sting = true, social = true, colour ≠ black. We must choose at least one item from the difference list. Note that we can not use the condition "striped", as this was also true for the cornerstone case. Therefore, this condition does not appear in the difference list. The node will be added as shown in Fig. 2. Our bee becomes the cornerstone case for node 4. Node 4 will now only fire in the same context as this case, i.e. after the same sequence of rules has fired.

Thus the core task for the expert is to find differences between sets of data (cases) that account for differences in interpretation. This task requires only domain expertise and is independent of KE.

Multiple-Classification Ripple-Down Rules

MC-RDR employ an n-ary, rather than a binary tree. Each node may have multiple children, and there is no "false" path structure. Each node is evaluated sequentially. If a node fires true, all of its children are also evaluated. If none of its children are true, then the conclusion for that node is generated for the case. The final output for a case is the sum of all of these conclusions that fire.

The core task for the expert (choosing conditions from difference lists and assigning interpretations) is essentially the same. However, there are some novel features of MC-RDR which impact upon the expert's task:

- Unlike RDR, where all corrections involve replacing a previous interpretation, the expert may either retain or suppress each interpretation generated. Any number of new interpretations may also be added.
- In RDR, new rules are always attached to the last node evaluated. For MC-RDR two options are available. Replacement rules qualify a previous rule, as in RDR. Top-level rules represent entirely new contexts. The nature of new rules needs to be identified by the expert.
- For suppressed conclusions which are not being replaced, stopping rules are needed. Stopping rules specify conditions under which a conclusion should not fire.
- MC-RDR nodes often have multiple cornerstone cases. Depending upon the conditions selected, the expert may be prompted to deal with a number of difference lists.

Programmes

A new interpreter, RDR Engine, was written in C. RDR Engine supports both MC-RDR and conventional RDR (hereafter referred to as RDR). The run time and maintenance environments were built as a Hypercard (Apple) stack.

All studies were performed using either Macintosh Quadra 840, LC630 or PowerBook 180c personal computers.

Evaluation of Multiple-Classification Ripple-Down Rules for Arterial Blood Gas Data

In order to compare MC-RDR with RDR, 262 cases with ABG data from the original PEIRS development were used. The same pathologist built knowledge bases for both MC-RDR and RDR from these cases. The cases were processed in the same sequence for both knowledge bases, with the same interpretative output constructed for each (for RDR: this required combining classifications into single comments, as for PEIRS). Data included pH, PCO_2, PO_2, calculated bicarbonate, base excess and patient's age on up to five sequential specimens.

The interpretative task was the diagnosis of disorders of acid–base balance and oxygen status. All cases were evaluated by a human expert, and the agreement between expert and ES was recorded. Accuracy was defined as the proportion of cases that agreed with the human expert's classification. The conclusion management screen is shown in Fig. 3.

Note that in Fig. 3 the system has produced five conclusions, two of which are deemed incorrect. The incorrect interpretations have been moved from the "current conclusions" box to the "deleted conclusions" box. One new interpretation has also been added. Three original interpretations are judged to be correct and remain in the "current conclusions" box. These conclusions need no further processing.

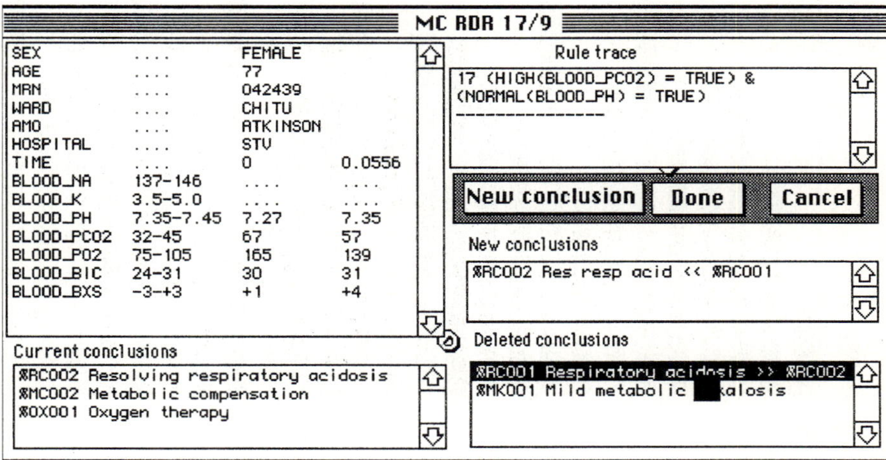

Fig. 3. Conclusion maintenance in multiple-classification ripple-down rules (MC-RDR). Note that conclusions can readily be moved between the "current conclusions" and "deleted conclusions" boxes. New conclusions may also be added

Results

Accuracy

The accuracy of the final systems, determined from the last 50 cases evaluated, was 84% for MC-RDR and 30% for RDR. Note that both knowledge bases were incomplete – mature knowledge bases would be expected to have more rules and a much greater accuracy. Most important for this study was not completeness, but the rate at which each system matured.

Maturation Rate

The maturation rate can be considered to be the rate at which the knowledge base develops towards acceptably accurate performance. MC-RDR matured much more quickly than RDR. Figures 4 and 5 show the development of recent accuracy (accuracy for the last ten cases evaluated) for each system.

Efficiency

Rules

Efficiency of KA is reflected in the rate of growth of the knowledge base and its overall size, compared with the accuracy of its performance. As shown

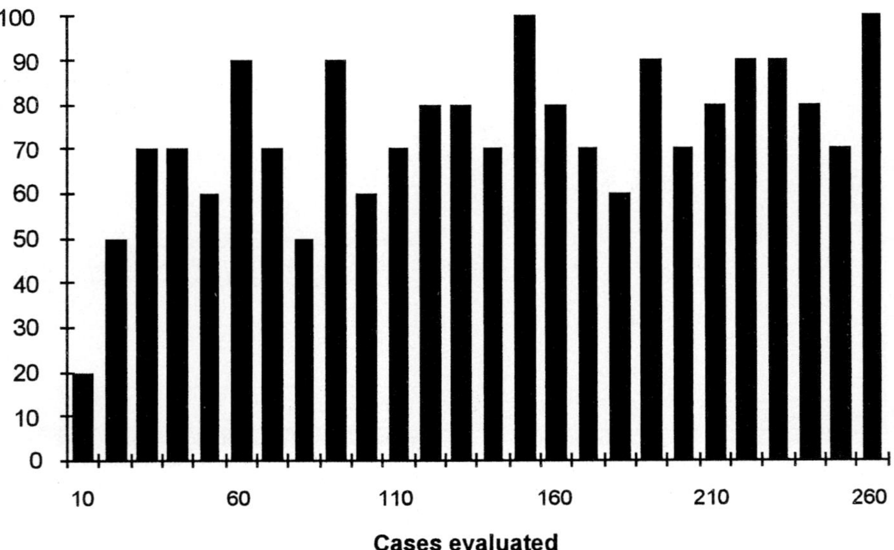

Fig. 4. Recent accuracy (last ten cases) for 262 cases processed with multiple-classification ripple-down rules (MC-RDR)

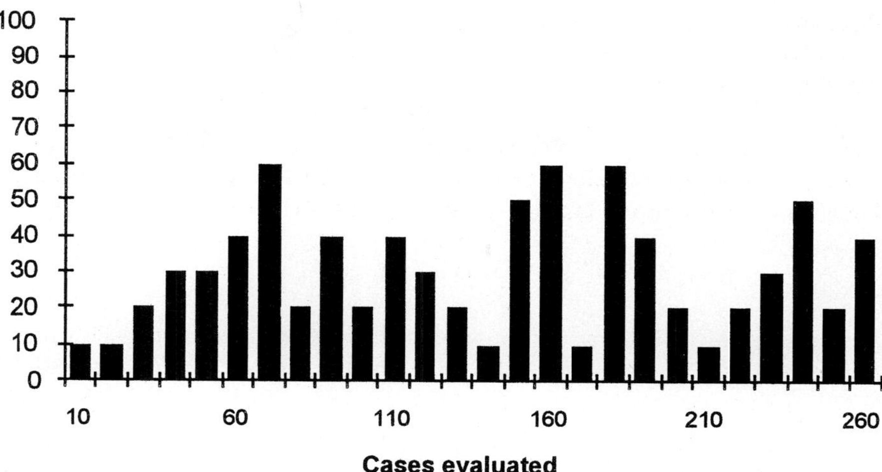

Fig. 5. Recent accuracy (last ten cases) for 262 cases processed with ripple-down rules (RDR)

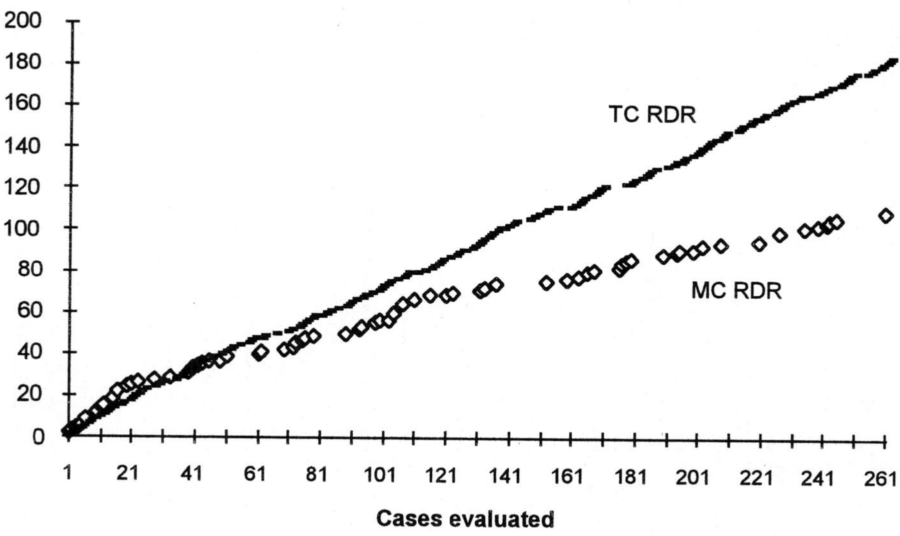

Fig. 6. Growth of knowledge base for multiple-classification ripple-down rules (*MC-RDR*) and RDR

above, MC-RDR achieved high accuracy much earlier than RDR. It also was far more efficient. Figure 6 compares the rate of knowledge base growth for the two systems.

RDR can be seen to be growing at a much greater rate than MC-RDR, except in the earliest phase (by definition, the maximum rate of growth for RDR is one rule per case; MC-RDR has no such limit). Compared to its high early growth rate, the growth rate of MC-RDR appears to be slowing, whereas there is no sign of this yet in RDR.

MC-RDR's final knowledge base contained 109 rules (262 rule conditions), in contrast to 184 rules (442 rule conditions) for RDR.

Conclusions

As expected, MC-RDR was far more efficient than RDR for conclusion management. After 262 cases, MC-RDR contained a total of 22 conclusions; 17 (77%) of these were re-used in more than one node. RDR contained 129 conclusions, with 39 (30%) re-used. This difference reflects the effort saved for the expert in building conclusions.

Invalid Combinations

As the final output of MC-RDR is a combination of individually generated conclusions, novel combinations will appear. In some instance, these were invalid. In Fig. 1, the system has produced both "respiratory acidosis" and "resolving respiratory acidosis." While both are true in a strict sense, the pathologist considered that these conclusions should not co-exist. In the current implementation, there was no mechanism for preventing invalid combinations.

Knowledge Maintenance Tasks

Dealing with multiple conclusions, rules and cornerstone cases made the expert's task, for individual cases, slightly more complex than for RDR. This had minimal impact upon the expert, however. Most notable for the expert was the substantial savings accruing from the vastly more compact and efficient knowledge base in MC-RDR, as shown above. A number of new issues for knowledge maintenance did arise, however.

Independence of Conclusions

Determining whether an interpretative statement is independent of the others is sometimes not clear-cut. There are instances in which conclusions are entirely unrelated (as in different domains), but for many others concepts may be related. For instance, the comment "Respiratory acidosis. Metabolic alkalosis" contains two such statements. These may well be co-existing disorders, originating from independently acquired disease processes. However, each impacts upon the measured pH, PCO_2 and PO_2, and the compensatory response to each disorder affects some of the same physiological systems. Thus, while each may occur alone, it is debatable whether their occurrence together should be considered as two separate disorders or a single entity, "mixed respiratory acidosis and metabolic alkalosis."

For this study, the expert chose to consider all disorders as discrete classifications, so that the above example would require two conclusions. In fact, he adopted a rather extreme approach, treating "metabolic compensation" as a discrete interpretation, even though it applies both to respiratory acidosis and alkalosis and is meaningless alone. This kept the number of interpretative comments stored in the system to a minimum and reduced the amount of work in maintaining conclusions. However, it probably increased the incidence of invalid combinations of conclusions.

Rule Management

The expert made considerable use of both replacement and top-level rules. As indicated earlier, this decision needed to be made by the expert. Deciding between replacement and top-level rules was usually straightforward, but occasionally the distinction was not clear-cut. Replacement rules were usually more attractive, as they minimised the work involved.

Discussion

This work has provided the first validation of MC-RDR in a multiple-classification domain. It has confirmed the compact nature of MC-RDR knowledge bases [16] and the far greater efficiency of KA compared with conventional RDR. Interpretative accuracy matures rapidly, supporting the incremental knowledge base development model established by PEIRS.

Interpretation of Arterial Blood Gas Data

ABG and acid–base status are subject to a range of pathological processes, several of which may co-exist. In addition, the severity and rapid progression of many disorders often warrants sequential analysis, so that data often contain a multitude of complex temporal trends. For this reason, a complex area was usually considered, requiring sophisticated modelling techniques for interpretation. A well-known system in this area is ABEL, which diagnoses disorders of acid–base and electrolyte physiology [10]. ABEL interprets only single data sets and is unable to deal with temporal trends. More recently, Coiera [11] has applied the QSIM qualitative modelling approach. This system uses "disease histories" to reason about the progression of acid–base disorders. Neither of these systems has ever seen routine operation. In contrast, MC-RDR supported the rapid development of an ABG ES, including temporal trends, without recourse to complex modelling.

Note that the evaluation commenced from the very first cases evaluated by each system, i.e. with empty knowledge bases. Accuracy at this stage of development would be expected to be low. In this sense, RDR's performance is possibly acceptable, given that it is a very "young" system. However, MC-RDR's performance was clearly vastly superior.

Temporal Data

The significance of temporal trends for ABG data is shown in Fig. 7. In this example, knowledge of previous data points to a likely *cause* for the metabolic alkalosis and substantially alters the management advice.

The ease with which temporal data was handled with MC-RDR contrasts with the conventional view that reasoning with temporal data is extremely complex [18] and challenges the notion that sophisticated domain modelling is required.

Knowledge Management

Local Knowledge

The ultimate success of MC-RDR in real-time interpretation in critical care settings will be determined by its acceptance by clinicians. While accuracy is important, acceptability will also depend upon the system's ability to reflect local practice, knowledge and beliefs.

As shown in Fig. 7, MC-RDR need not be restricted to diagnosis. As with PEIRS, therapeutic or test ordering advice can readily be implemented. This sort of management advice tends to be even more subject to local protocol than diagnosis. Readily supportable by MC-RDR, these local protocols would be very difficult to maintain with conventional ES technology.

For individual cases, local knowledge maintenance with MC-RDR was only marginally more complex than for conventional RDR. A number of minor issues, such as the ambiguity over independence of conclusions, complicated the task slightly. However, these were more than offset by the elimination of the multiple-classification problem. The overall maintenance workload was substantially reduced in MC-RDR, evidenced by the highly compact knowledge base. Further work is underway to resolve the issues of top-level versus replacement rules and the ambiguity of independent conclusions.

Clinical Data

Meaningful interpretation is clearly dependant upon the clinical context in which tests are performed. Computers will never be able to capture the wealth of clinical knowledge available to clinicians, and computers will therefore always support, rather than replace, human experts. In this study, no

```
SEX  ....  MALE
AGE  ....  44
WARD ....  CHITU
HOSPITAL ....  STV
TIME ....  0
BLOOD_pH 7.35--7.45  7.51
BLOOD_PCO2  32--45 39
BLOOD_PO2 75--105 87
BLOOD_BIC 24--31 31
BLOOD_BXS -3-+3 +8
```

Results consistent with: Metabolic alkalosis.

Suggest: Attend to cause, including fluid losses & diuretic therapy. Check serum potassium level. Repeat ABGs to monitor progress.

```
SEX  ....  MALE
AGE  ....  44
WARD ....  CHITU
HOSPITAL ....  STV
TIME ....  0  0.0465  0.5444  0.7451  1.023
BLOOD_pH 7.35--7.45  7.27  ....  7.35 7.37 7.51
BLOOD_PCO2  32--45 67  ....  57 52 39
BLOOD_PO2 75--105 115  ....  120 119 87
BLOOD_BIC 24--31 30  ....  31 30 31
BLOOD_BXS -3-+3 +1  ....  +4 +4 +8
```

Results consistent with: Resolution of respiratory acidosis. Post-hypercapnoeic metabolic alkalosis.

Suggest: Ensure adequate hydration & renal function. No action required.

Fig. 7. Impact of access to temporal trends on diagnosis and management advice. Interpretation with and without previous data is shown. Note: therapeutic advice comments, added here for illustration, were not included in PEIRS. *BIC*, Bicarbonate; *BXS*, base excess

clinical data other than patient's age was available. Other data, such as FiO_2, clinical history and results of other investigations, would obviously enhance the quality of the interpretation. However, some value can always be added to raw data in the absence of clinical information, as in the detection of significant disorders of acid–base status. Access to more detailed clinical data for an ABG ES will require either user input (such as FiO_2) or interfaces to other information systems. In the meantime, however, clinically useful interpretation can be achieved with a minimum of clinical data.

We have shown that MC-RDR removes the constraints that the multiple-classification problem imposed on PEIRS. An ES for interpreting ABG data, including temporal trends, has been built by a domain expert without KA support or skills. The knowledge base matured rapidly and would be suitable for incorporation into analytical instruments in critical care. Further work should clarify the need for replacement and top-level rules. The problem of invalid combinations of conclusions is also being addressed. Tools to help experts determine the most appropriate contents of classifications, especially with regard to combined versus discrete interpretations, may also be needed.

We believe that, combined with an effective error management strategy, locally managed MC-RDR ES will improve the utility of decision support tools in critical care. Manufacturers might embed MC-RDR ES into their analytical instruments' software and assist in distributing knowledge base updates. A knowledge maintenance application may reside on a senior clinician's desktop computer, enabling modifications to be added as required. Interpretative comments incorporating local knowledge will not only support patient care decisions, but will contribute to the education of junior medical and other clinical staff. Most importantly, simple and rapid localisation of knowledge bases by senior clinicians will enable systems to remain current and relevant to local practice.

Acknowledgments. This work is supported in part by the Australian Research Council. Dr. Edwards is supported by a Medical Post-Graduate Research Scholarship from the New South Wales Department of Health.

References

1. Leape L (1994) Error in medicine. JAMA 272:1851–1857
2. Coiera E (1993) Informatics – the future of laboratory medicine. Oral communication. Presented at the XV International Congress of Clinical Chemistry, Uluru, Australia, 22–24 November
3. Barro S, Presedo J, Vila J, Ruiz R, Palacios F (1993) Patient management in CCUs: need for an intelligent interpretation of signals. Expert Systems Appl 6:421–432
4. Coiera E (1993) Intelligent monitoring and control of dynamic physiological systems. Artif Intell Med 5:1–8
5. Haug P, Gardner R, Tate K et al (1994) Decision support in medicine: examples from the HELP system. Comput Biomed Res 27:396–418
6. Johnston M, Langton K, Haynes R, Mathieu A (1994) Effects of computer-based clinical decision support systems on clinician performance and patient outcome. Ann Intern Med 120:135–142
7. Tierney W, Hui S, McDonald C (1986) Delayed feedback of physician performance versus immediate reminders to perform preventative care. Med Care 24:659
8. Shapiro B (1995) Clinical and economic performance criteria for intraarterial and extraarterial blood gas monitors, with comparison with in vitro testing. Am J Clin Pathol 104:S100-S106
9. Bleich H (1972) Computer-based consultation: electrolyte and acid-base disorders. Am J Med 53:285–291
10. Patil R, Szolovits P, Schwartz W (1982) Modelling knowledge of the patient in acid-base and electrolyte disorders. In: Szolovits P (ed) Artificial intelligence in medicine. Westview, Boulder, pp 191–226
11. Coiera E (1989) Reasoning with qualitative disease histories for diagnostic patient monitoring. Ph.D. Thesis, University of New South Wales

12. Gaines B, Shaw M (1991) Foundations of knowledge acquisition. In: Motoda H, Mizoguchi R, Boose J, Gaines B (eds) Knowledge acquisition for knowledge-based systems. Ohmsha, Tokyo, pp 3–24
13. Compton P, Jansen R (1990) A philosophical basis for knowledge acquisition. Knowledge Acquisition 2:241–257
14. Edwards G, Srinivasan A, Compton P, Malor R, Lazarus L (1991) A user-maintained expert system for the interpretation of chemical pathology reports. Clin Biochem Rev 12:66
15. Clancey W (1995) The learning process in the epistemology of medical information. Methods Inform Med 34:122–130
16. Kang BH, Compton P, Preston P (1995) Multiple classification ripple down rules: evaluation and possibilities. In: Gaines BR, Musen M (eds) 9th Knowledge Acquisition for Knowledge Based Systems Workshop. SRDG Publications, Banff, pp 17.1–17.20
17. Kang B (1995) Validating knowledge acquisition: multiple classifications ripple down rules. Ph.D. Thesis, University of New South Wales
18. Leng W, Pau L (1991) Temporal reasoning in blood gas analysis. Expert Systems 8:159–170

Computer-Assisted Evaluation
of Oxygen and Acid–Base Status of the Blood

M. Siggaard-Andersen

Abstract

More than ten standard equations describing physiological dependencies of blood oxygen and acid–base status were combined with the TANH equation to model the haemoglobin oxygen-binding curve in a computer programme called the Oxygen Status Algorithm. The programme takes measured quantities from blood gas analysers and multi-wavelength spectrophotometers together with a few user-supplied values to calculate a number of derived quantities. The resulting comprehensive blood gas analysis contains almost 30 values, which may be combined, displayed and interpreted with the aid of the programme. It is possible to test the effects of therapeutic measures using "what if" functions, reversing several of the calculations. On-line versions are being developed for several commercial analysers allowing easy collection of data. A new interface based on the Windows environment is discussed that makes almost exclusive use of graphical solutions for presentation of the results and interaction with the user.

Introduction

This paper describes a computer programme for calculation and display of the oxygen status and the acid–base status of the blood. The purpose of the programme is to enhance the benefit of measuring arterial and mixed-venous blood gas data, aiding in the interpretation and making the complex relationships comprehensible even to less experienced physicians. This is relevant when advanced blood gas analytical instruments become more widespread and are placed under supervision in departments with expertise in areas other than pH and blood gas disorders. With the large number of measured and derived quantities presented by modern analytical instruments, users may be tempted to disregard most of these and focus their attention on as few as two or three "key" quantities, the interpretation of which may still be difficult. Moreover, the previous use of nomograms emphasized the relationship between quantities, interdependencies which are far from obvious in today's numerical output. For the same reasons, assistance in selecting treatments is also desirable.

One solution to the above-mentioned problems is to use artificial intelligence or learning-based systems to cope with the number crunching and to suggest a diagnosis and treatment. However, this could make it difficult to predict or reconstruct decision making by the algorithm. In the case of blood pH and blood gases, the physiological relationships are well described and can at least be accurately modelled. We have thus attempted to solve the problems by classical programming techniques and to calculate the effects of various treatments by reversal of the mathematical procedures.

Programming of the Oxygen Status Algorithm began several years ago during development of the TANH equation for the haemoglobin–oxygen affinity curve [1]. The latter allowed us to accurately model the relationship between the oxygen partial pressure and the oxygen saturation fraction of human blood, taking the Bohr effect, temperature and concentration of 2,3-diphosphoglycerate in erythrocytes into account. Together with a number of well-described physiological relationships, the TANH equation was placed at the centre of a computer programme to handle the more than 30 measured and calculated quantities that constitute a comprehensive pH and blood gas analysis. This programme has evolved from a simple algorithm to test the applicability of the TANH equation into the present versions that feature on-line data collection from commercial analysers, several graphical displays aiding interpretation and printed reports with appropriately calculated reference intervals.

Materials and Methods

Data

Measured Values

A modern pH blood gas analyser measures pH, PCO_2 and PO_2, while the haemoximeter provides values for oxygen saturation, carboxyhaemoglobin, methaemoglobin, and total haemoglobin.

Supplementary Data

The above-mentioned values are supplemented by patient temperature, inspired oxygen fraction, fraction of fetal haemoglobin and ambient pressure to allow all the calculations to be carried out. The programme provides appropriately calculated reference values when the patient's age and sex is entered.

Calculated Values

Of the many parameters that can be calculated and presented, we have chosen the most significant: inspired and alveolar oxygen partial pressures, pH,

PCO_2 and PO_2 referring to the actual patient temperature, estimated shunt fraction, half-saturation tension, estimated 2,3-diphosphoglycerate concentration, oxygen capacity and content, extracellular base excess and plasma bicarbonate concentration.

To quantitate the combined effects of the arterial oxygen tension, effective haemoglobin concentration and half saturation tension, a new quantity named the oxygen extraction tension (px) was introduced [6]. It is defined as the tension obtained after extracting 2.3 mmol oxygen/l from arterial blood and is calculated on the basis of the mathematical model of the blood oxygen-binding curve for the patient. The resulting oxygen partial pressure can readily be compared with that required for maintenance of an adequate O_2 gradient to the mitochondrion.

Equations

Ten equations are at the core of the programme:
1.   The TANH equation to describe the oxygen dissociation curve [1, 2]
2.   The Haldane equation for carbon monoxide binding
3.   The Henderson-Hasselbalch equation, which expresses pH as a function of bicarbonate and PCO_2
4.   The Van Slyke equation for base excess [5]
5.   The total oxygen equation, which combines soluble and haeme-bound oxygen
6.   The alveolar air equation, which calculates the alveolar oxygen partial pressure from that of the inspired air, PCO_2 and the respiratory quotient [7]
7.   The shunt equation, which expresses the fraction of venous blood shunted past the alveoles
8–10. The temperature coefficients for pH, PCO_2 and PO_2

Programming

Hard- and Software Platform

At the time of development, MS-DOS version 2.11 was the dominating operating system chosen as the platform for the distributed versions 2.X and 3.X of the Oxygen Status Algorithm. The only additional requirement added to those for running DOS was a 512-kB RAM configuration. We used Turbo Pascal version 5.5 (Borland International, Scotts Valley, CA) as the programming language and the Object Professional Toolbox (Turbo Power Software, Scotts Valley, CA) to provide a tested code for all standard tasks.

Support for VGA, EGA, CGA and Hercules graphical displays and for Epson 8-pin and HP Laserjet series II printers was included in version 2.X. Later, Epson 24-pin and IBM printers were added, while no updates have been made to the list of supported displays. Using DOS, the work load for coding the display and printer support has been out of proportion with its significance for the usability of the algorithms.

A new version of the programme written for a modern graphically operating environment has been underway for some time. In this version, most of the problems associated with display and printer support will be offloaded from our programme and handled by the operating system. We have chosen Windows for this development. Several working models have been coded, using Visual Basic (Microsoft), Turbo Pascal for Windows and Delphi (Borland). As discussed later, some of the planned graphics functions require rapid recalculations and redrawing of the screen images. Thus a compiled language will be chosen for the final version, and we may use the new "games developers toolkit" to allow the fast, smooth, real-time redraws characteristic of computer games in our interactive graphics solutions.

Error Handling

Early in the development, it became apparent that it was difficult to predict whether all equations could be solved with any given data set. Although great care was taken in testing the parameters before passing them on to the core procedures, there was no way to ensure that no errors could arise in these calculations. We implemented a routine to trap the "exception interrupts" generated by the 80XXX series microprocessors upon internal calculational errors and were thus able to take control after events such as divide by zero or logarithm of a negative number. The user cannot distinguish between this kind of error handling and that taking place in explicit programme statements; both result in the message "unable to calculate (current case)".

In each part of the programme, an "exit procedure" is defined, which is placed in a chain executed upon programme termination. Statements in these blocks are carried out even after most kinds of programme crash and provide a neat way of cleaning up and making sure that data files are properly written and closed, for example.

The resulting algorithm has been extremely stable, and to our knowledge it has not caused any errors or data loss over several years of use.

The Programme

Data Input–Output Screen

The Oxygen Status Algorithm is built around a main data input–output screen which contains all the measured and calculated quantities (Fig. 1). Patient information and a short user-defined comment are placed at the top of the screen, while an area for help and error messages is found in the bottom right-hand corner. Rather than simply grouping the quantities into columns

```
 ID: Case 1 (first sample)      # 1   | Chronic obstructive lung disease
 Arterial blood from male  , age 61 y | Pickwick syndrome
 Sample date 91-01-07, time 11:40     | /R
 ------------------------------------ | ------------------------------------
    pressure            Units:        |    conc            Units:
 TPt          37.2         °C         |    ctHb + 9.7        mmol/L
       Pamb +101.3    kPa             | FCOHb          1.0           %
 FO2dI        80.0*        %          | FMetHb         0.9           %
       pO2hI + 76.0*   kPa            |    ceHb + 9.5        mmol/L
 RQ           0.86         1          | sO2a          96.7*          %
 pCO2a        5.7          kPa        |    ctO2 + 9.3        mmol/L
       pO2A + 70.0*   kPa             |    cO2Hb + 9.2       mmol/L
 Fva          29.*         %          |
       pO2a + 11.8    kPa             |                :
         px + 5.1     kPa             | FHbF     :    0.5            %
 pHa          7.49*        1          | ------------------------------------
        p50 + 3.5     kPa             |  cBaseEcf :  8.4*     mmol/L
 cDPG    :    6.1*     mmol/L         |  cHCO3(P) : 32.2*     mmol/L
 ------------------------------------ | ------------------------------------
 T meas.   :    37.0       °C         | Enter name or ID for patient. Use
    pO2(37) :11.63     kPa            | ENTER to accept, ESC to cancel
 pCO2(37)  :     5.69      kPa        | changes, or ↑↓←→ to move to other
 pH(37)    :     7.491*    1          | fields.
                                      --- Oxygen Status Algorithm V3.UK-95 ---
```

Fig. 1. The data input–output screen of the Oxygen Status Algorithm. On the computer screen, different colours are used to distinguish between instrument input, user input and calculated values. Columns containing the units of measure may be switched to show either reference intervals or the source of the value. *Asterisks* next to values are coded red or blue and indicate a value over or below the reference interval, respectively. The case shown was taken from the examples included with the programme

of input and output parameters, care was taken to group the parameters to reflect their physiological relationships.

Pressure-Related Parameters

The middle left-hand panel contains parameters relating to the oxygen partial pressure placed along a scale starting with ambient pressure and displaying all the oxygen tensions in decreasing order. Interposed along the scale are those quantities which determine each drop in oxygen tension along the scale.

Concentration-Related Parameters

The right-hand panel shows a scale with the haemoglobin and oxygen concentrations from total haemoglobin to effective haemoglobin down to oxyhaemoglobin. Again, the values quantitating each drop along the scale are found interposed.

Acid–Base-Related Parameters

One of the most important acid–base parameters, pH, is shown in connection with the half-saturation tension P_{50}, which it influences due to the Bohr effect. Similarly, PCO_2 is interposed on the pressure scale because of its influence on the decrease in PO_2 from inspired to alveolar air.

Graphs and Interpretation

The programme can present the data of the input–output screen in a number of different ways to enhance their perception.

pH Chart

The pH graph illustrates the relationship between the dependent variable pH and the two independent variables pCO_2 and the base excess of the extracellular fluid. The latter is recognized as being the most relevant measure of a non-respiratory (metabolic) acid–base disturbance. Reference areas for this and other classes of acid–base disturbances are indicated on the graph (Fig. 2, top right) [10]. When viewing the three quantities in terms of dependent and independent variables, the offset of pH from the normal 7.4 can be seen as a lack of compensation.

O_2 Graph

A graph with a logarithmic PO_2 scale as the abscissa and a concentration scale as the ordinate is used to display the modelled oxygen-binding curve (Fig. 2, top left). Note that these scales are the same as those used in the left- and right-hand panels of the data input–output screen and that the displayed quantities are the same. However, when put on a graph, the correspondence between values becomes much more apparent and the user is forced to view and consider all available parameters.

Haemoglobin concentrations are shown along the left scale and affect the "height" of the curve along with the maximum obtainable oxygen concentrations indicated at the right ordinate. Once the curve has been constructed, markers are added along the pressure gradient from ambient pressure, to inspired oxygen tension, to partial pressure of oxygen in the alveole to the oxygen tension in arterial blood. From this point, a bold arrow follows the curve, indicating the extraction of 2.3 mmol oxygen/l, ending at the point defined as the oxygen extraction tension, px. Finally, P_{50} and its offset from the standard value is shown, indicating the horizontal shift of the curve.

The oxygen extraction tension px depends upon the three physiologically independent quantities PO_2, ceHb, and P_{50}. A normal px of about 5 kPa thus indicates that the three quantities on which it depends are either all normal or that compensation has taken place. In turn, this eases interpretation of combined changes in the three independent parameters.

The oxygen graph and acid–base charts together constitute a complete pH and blood gas analysis and may allow the most intuitive interpretation. We have thus tested the possibility of basing the entire reporting on graphs, on which exact values for every quantity may be obtained by simple pointing with a mouse. The results obtained are quite promising and have led to further developments of this concept, as discussed below.

The Oxygen Status Algorithm: Patient Status Report.   Oxygen & Acid-Base Status of the Blood.

Pt.ID: Case 1 (first sample)	Sample Date: 91-01-07	Comment: Chronic obstructive lung disease
male	Sample time: 11:40	Pickwick syndrome
age 61 years	Arterial blood	/R

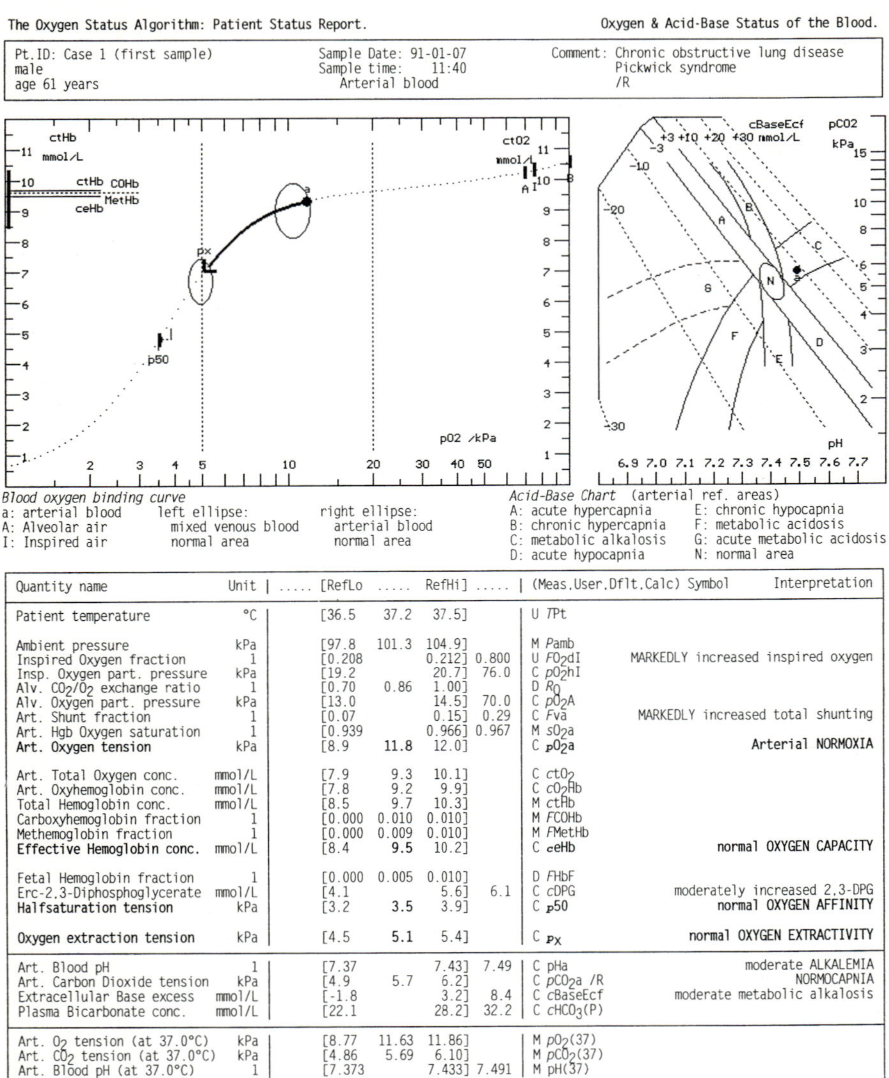

Blood oxygen binding curve
a: arterial blood   left ellipse: right ellipse:
A: Alveolar air   mixed venous blood   arterial blood
I: Inspired air   normal area   normal area

Acid-Base Chart (arterial ref. areas)
A: acute hypercapnia   E: chronic hypocapnia
B: chronic hypercapnia   F: metabolic acidosis
C: metabolic alkalosis   G: acute metabolic acidosis
D: acute hypocapnia   N: normal area

Quantity name	Unit	[RefLo	.....	RefHi]	.....	(Meas.User.Dflt.Calc) Symbol	Interpretation
Patient temperature	°C	[36.5	37.2	37.5]		U TPt	
Ambient pressure	kPa	[97.8	101.3	104.9]		M Pamb	
Inspired Oxygen fraction	1	[0.208		0.212]	0.800	U FO$_2$dI	MARKEDLY increased inspired oxygen
Insp. Oxygen part. pressure	kPa	[19.2		20.7]	76.0	C pO$_2$hI	
Alv. CO$_2$/O$_2$ exchange ratio	1	[0.70	0.86	1.00]		D R_0	
Alv. Oxygen part. pressure	kPa	[13.0		14.5]	70.0	C pO$_2$A	
Art. Shunt fraction	1	[0.07		0.15]	0.29	C Fva	MARKEDLY increased total shunting
Art. Hgb Oxygen saturation	1	[0.939		0.966]	0.967	M sO$_2$a	
Art. Oxygen tension	kPa	[8.9	**11.8**	12.0]		C $_p$O$_2$a	Arterial NORMOXIA
Art. Total Oxygen conc.	mmol/L	[7.9	9.3	10.1]		C ctO$_2$	
Art. Oxyhemoglobin conc.	mmol/L	[7.8	9.2	9.9]		C cO$_2$Hb	
Total Hemoglobin conc.	mmol/L	[8.5	9.7	10.3]		M ctHb	
Carboxyhemoglobin fraction	1	[0.000	0.010	0.010]		M FCOHb	
Methemoglobin fraction	1	[0.000	0.009	0.010]		M FMetHb	
Effective Hemoglobin conc.	mmol/L	[8.4	**9.5**	10.2]		C ceHb	normal OXYGEN CAPACITY
Fetal Hemoglobin fraction	1	[0.000	0.005	0.010]		D FHbF	
Erc-2.3-Diphosphoglycerate	mmol/L	[4.1		5.6]	6.1	C cDPG	moderately increased 2.3-DPG
Halfsaturation tension	kPa	[3.2	**3.5**	3.9]		C $_p$50	normal OXYGEN AFFINITY
Oxygen extraction tension	kPa	[4.5	**5.1**	5.4]		C $_p$X	normal OXYGEN EXTRACTIVITY
Art. Blood pH	1	[7.37		7.43]	7.49	C pHa	moderate ALKALEMIA
Art. Carbon Dioxide tension	kPa	[4.9	5.7	6.2]		C pCO$_2$a /R	NORMOCAPNIA
Extracellular Base excess	mmol/L	[-1.8		3.2]	8.4	C cBaseEcf	moderate metabolic alkalosis
Plasma Bicarbonate conc.	mmol/L	[22.1		28.2]	32.2	C cHCO$_3$(P)	
Art. O$_2$ tension (at 37.0°C)	kPa	[8.77	11.63	11.86]		M pO$_2$(37)	
Art. CO$_2$ tension (at 37.0°C)	kPa	[4.86	5.69	6.10]		M pCO$_2$(37)	
Art. Blood pH (at 37.0°C)	1	[7.373		7.433]	7.491	M pH(37)	

Reference: Siggaard-Andersen, Mads & Siggaard-Andersen, Ole.
Oxygen status algorithm, version 3, with some applications. Acta Anaesth Scand 1995; 39, Suppl. 107: 13-20.

Fig. 2. Printed status report produced by the Oxygen Status Algorithm, version 3. It illustrates the layout of the pH chart, oxygen graph and numerical results with reference values and verbal interpretation

Gas Map

The relationship between the arterial blood gases is illustrated in a graph with PO$_2$ on the abscissa and the PCO$_2$ on the ordinate, both on logarithmic scales [8, 9]. From the reference area for arterial blood, the relationship between PO_2 and PCO_2 resulting from primary changes in PO_2 or PCO_2 is indicated (see Fig. 4 in [3] for a printed example of this graph type).

Laboratory Diagnosis

As an aid in interpreting the numbers presented on the data input–output screen, a verbal "laboratory diagnosis" may be displayed (Fig. 3). This uses a set of arbitrary levels to classify each quantity as being either normal or slightly, moderately, markedly, or extremely elevated or decreased. The top part displays a report on arterial oxygen status, divided into sections corresponding to the three physiologically independent quantities PO_2, ceHb and P_{50}. For each quantity, the quantities upon which they depend may be specified when they deviate from what is considered normal. The oxygen status is summarized in a single line, based on the calculated value for the oxygen extraction tension, px. The acid–base status shown at the bottom of the diagnosis screen is classified according to pH as acidaemia, neutralaemia or alkalaemia, with the underlying respiratory or metabolic disturbances indicated.

Help System

The present DOS versions incorporate a comprehensive context-sensitive help system covering both the programme's function and physiological theory. Future versions written for the Windows help programme will benefit from the graphical environment. The readability will be enhanced by correct display of units and symbols using italic, super and subscript type and of equations,

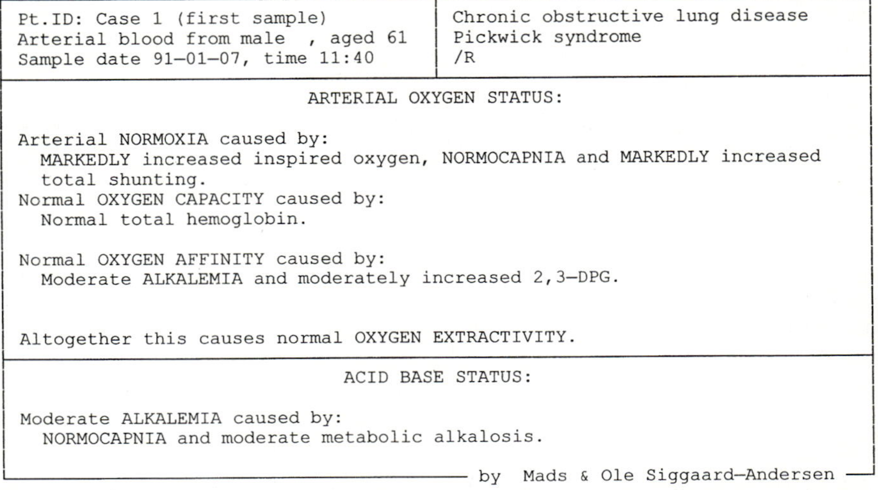

```
Pt.ID: Case 1 (first sample)     Chronic obstructive lung disease
Arterial blood from male  , aged 61   Pickwick syndrome
Sample date 91-01-07, time 11:40     /R

                    ARTERIAL OXYGEN STATUS:

Arterial NORMOXIA caused by:
  MARKEDLY increased inspired oxygen, NORMOCAPNIA and MARKEDLY increased
  total shunting.
Normal OXYGEN CAPACITY caused by:
  Normal total hemoglobin.

Normal OXYGEN AFFINITY caused by:
  Moderate ALKALEMIA and moderately increased 2,3-DPG.


Altogether this causes normal OXYGEN EXTRACTIVITY.

                     ACID BASE STATUS:

Moderate ALKALEMIA caused by:
  NORMOCAPNIA and moderate metabolic alkalosis.
                           by  Mads & Ole Siggaard-Andersen
```

Fig. 3. The verbal "laboratory diagnosis," interpreting the arterial pH and blood gas analysis

as a result of dedicated editors. The addition of graphs and explanatory pictures may allow the help system to develop into an on-line physiological textbook. In turn, one may envisage the programme providing help from this "textbook", depending on the kind of user, i.e. technician, scientist or student.

Printed Output

Status Report

The printed status report incorporates parts from the data input–output screen, the laboratory diagnosis and the graphical displays (Fig. 2). To allow quick identification of abnormal values, the results appear in three columns placed relative to their reference values. Each quantity is interpreted in terms of the previously described laboratory diagnosis. At the top of the printout, the oxygen graph and acid–base chart are included.

Cumulative Report

For records stored under identical patient identifications, a printout of key quantities ordered in reverse chronological order may be obtained. This is useful when monitoring a patient over time and allows quick identification of changing quantities.

Interfacing

On-Line Capability

On-line data collection from commercial analysers is possible in several versions of the Oxygen Status Algorithm distributed for research purposes. The experience gathered over several years of use in an intensive care unit is good and prompted the recent implementation of support for additional popular analysers.

Data File

The initial programme versions used an internal format for storing the patient data, but it quickly became apparent that some way of sharing data with other applications was desirable. At that time, a limitation in the number of fields per patient record precluded the use of a commercial database format for DOS. Thus the standard spreadsheet file format, as defined by Lotus Development (*.WK1 format), was chosen. This allowed most spreadsheet programmes to open the data files and perform further calculations and statistical evaluations outside the worksheet area used by our programme. It also became possible to enter data through this file and thus perform calculations on a large number of existing real or artificial patient cases in a batchwise mode.

The data format used by future programme versions has not yet been decided upon, although the close integration of routines to handle database records in the evaluated programming languages makes a database approach most likely. The need to store historical data for current patients and to collect long-term data for later identification of interesting cases or statistical evaluation also points toward a solution based on database records.

Data Exchange

As laboratory data systems become more advanced and electronic patient records more widespread, a version which works solely within other applications may be developed. By incorporating the Oxygen Status Algorithm as an object linking and embedding (OLE) server or exchanging data by dynamic data exchange (DDE), the programme will work seamlessly with other applications, providing its calculational, graphical and predictive powers. This will allow us to concentrate our work on the core of the algorithm within our area of expertise and to let the server application provide all the other support, including data storage and retrieval capabilities.

Discussion

Although modern blood gas analysers essentially calculate the same derived quantities as does the Oxygen Status Algorithm, the latter guides the user much better in understanding and interpreting the results. This is achieved by a physiologically relevant ordering of results and by graphic presentations to view the relationships between quantities and their combined effect on the patient acid–base and oxygen status. Interpretation of the results is also aided by calculation of relevant reference values for each patient.

While all of the above could be easily implemented on any blood gas analyser, some other features are currently only available with the Oxygen Status Algorithm. One is the ability to combine the results of two measurements, one from arterial and one from mixed venous blood. This allows more accurate calculations of the shunt fraction and CO_2/O_2 exchange ratio (RQ). Furthermore, if the cardiac output is known, the programme will determine the oxygen consumption rate, seen by some as the ultimate oxygen parameter.

Another feature specific to the Oxygen Status Algorithm is the ability to reverse the calculations and to provide a "what if" function. Once the relevant quantities have been determined for the patient's present situation, the predicted effect of several therapeutic measures may be easily tested. While this currently requires the user to specify the calculation mode and to modify values using the data input–output screen, models of the programme in which the "what if" function works in a graphical mode have been made. Using a pointing device, i.e. a mouse, the physician may take a marker from one of the graphs and drag it to the desired location. This action is immediately reflected in the calculations, and the graphs are continuously redrawn to allow very rapid determination of the optimal treatment. Verbal reports such as "the oxygen availability may be changed from markedly to moderately decreased by changing the oxygen tension of inspired air from 20 to 80 kPa" could be easily generated.

Three years of experience using continuous on-line operation of the programme in the intensive care unit have indicated that the programme assists the physician in decision making and have shown that the programme is very robust in routine use. As a teaching aid, the Oxygen Status Algorithm has been very useful in explaining the complex relationships of human respiratory physiology.

Conclusions

With the Oxygen Status Algorithm, we have provided a tool for comprehensive analysis of blood gas and pH measurements, with an emphasis on the underlying physiology. It is useful when carrying out calculations, interpretations or treatments and for teaching the relationships between the many quantities. The present versions of the programme are freely available from the authors for use in teaching and for performing scientific studies.

Acknowledgements. The programme described was developed in close collaboration with Professor O. Siggaard-Andersen, Department of Clinical Biochemistry, Herlev Hospital, DK-2730 Herlev. Support, suggestions and testing provided by Dr. I.H. Gøthgen (Department of Anaesthesia and Intensive Therapy, Gentofte Hospital, DK-2900 Hellerup, Denmark) are gratefully acknowledged.

References

1. Siggaard-Andersen O, Wimberley PD, Gøthgen IH, Siggaard-Andersen M (1984) A mathematical model of the hemoglobin-oxygen dissociation curve of human blood and of the oxygen partial pressure as a function of temperature. Clin Chem 30:1646–1651
2. Siggaard-Andersen O, Siggaard-Andersen M, Fogh-Andersen N (1993) The TANH equation modified for the hemoglobin, oxygen and carbon monoxide equilibrium. Scand J Clin Lab Invest 53 [Suppl 214]:113–119
3. Siggaard-Andersen O, Siggaard-Andersen M (1990) The oxygen status algorithm: a computer program for calculating and displaying pH and blood gas data. Scand J Clin Lab Invest 50 [Suppl 203]:29–45
4. Siggaard-Andersen M, Siggaard-Andersen O (1995) Oxygen status algorithm, version 3, with some applications. Acta Anaesth Scand 39 [Suppl 107]:13–20
5. Siggaard-Andersen O (1977) The Van Slyke equation. Scand J Clin Lab Invest Suppl 146:15–20
6. Siggaard-Andersen O, Gøthgen IH, Wimberley PD, Fogh-Andersen N (1990) The oxygen status of the arterial blood revised: relevant oxygen parameters for monitoring the arterial oxygen availablility. Scand J Clin Lab Invest 50 [Suppl 203]:17–28

7. Siggaard-Andersen O, Wimberley PD, Fogh-Andersen N, Gøthgen IH (1988) Measured and derived quantities with modern pH and blood gas equipment: calculation algorithms with 54 equations. Scand J Clin Lab Invest [Suppl 189]:7–15

8. Siggaard-Andersen O (1979) Hydrogen ions and blood gases. In: Brown SS, Mitchell FL, Young DS (eds) Chemical diagnosis of disease. Elsevier, Amsterdam, pp 181–245

9. Siggaard-Andersen O (1980) Determination and presentation of acid-base data. Contr Nephrol 21:128–136

10. Siggaard-Andersen O (1971) An acid-base chart for arterial blood with normal and pathophysiological reference areas. Scand J Clin Lab Invest 27:239–245

Pattern of Ionised Versus Total Magnesium Concentration in Peri-Operative Cardiac Surgery Patients: Influence of Preoperative Diuretic Therapy

I. Leonard, J. Collier, S. Maguire, D. Phelan, J. Fitzgerald, and B. Harte

Introduction

Previous studies have shown that levels of total magnesium are often low in peri-operative cardiac patients [1]. Because ionised magnesium has been advanced as a superior physiological indicator of magnesium status, we measured ionised magnesium in patients undergoing cardiac surgery to reassess the incidence of hypomagnesaemia in these patients.

Materials and Methods

Ionised and total magnesium measurements were made on 36 patients undergoing cardiopulmonary bypass, all of whom received standard cardioplegia solution intra-operatively (16 mmol magnesium chloride per l). Eleven patients were on diuretic therapy preoperatively, and 27 patients acted as controls. Samples were taken preoperatively and 1, 5 and 12 h postoperatively. Ionised magnesium, corrected for pH, was measured on a Nova Stat Profile 8 analyser (reference range, 0.42–0.60 mmol/l), and total magnesium was measured on a Beckman Synchron CX7 (reference range, 0.70–1.00 mmol/l).

Results

Table 1 shows the total and ionised magnesium results in each time group for the diuretic and control patient groups. The overall incidence of hypomagnesaemia, as measured by total and ionised magnesium, was low (2.7%) preoperatively, but increased to 16.6% at 12 h postoperatively. The mean total magnesium was significantly different between the two groups, both preoperatively and at 1 h postoperatively ($p<0.05$, Wilcoxon's test). There was no significant difference at any time in ionised magnesium between the two groups, and the only patients who had ionised hypomagnesaemia were in the diuretic group.

Table 1. Total and ionised magnesium results in diuretic and control patient groups (mean±SD)

Time	Total magnesium (mmol/l)[a]		Ionised magnesium (mmol/l)[b]	
	Diuretics	Control	Diuretics	Control
Preoperative	0.85±0.14	0.86±0.07	0.48±0.06	0.50±0.04
1 h postoperative	1.17±0.18	1.01±0.18	0.67±0.28	0.61±0.11
5 h postoperative	1.05±0.23	0.91±0.30	0.56±0.10	0.58±0.15
12 h postoperative	0.92±0.19	0.76±0.11	0.58±0.18	0.53±0.08

[a] Reference range, 0.70–1.00 mmol/l.
[b] Reference range, 0.42–0.60 mmol/l.

Conclusions

We conclude from this study that the incidence of ionised hypomagnesaemia is less common than previously reported for total magnesium measurements, and fluctuations in total magnesium are not reflected in ionised magnesium. Further studies will be undertaken to define the incidence of ionised hypomagnesaemia in diuretic patients undergoing cardiac surgery.

References

1. Aglio LS, Stanford GG, Maddi R et al. (1991) Hypomagnasaemia is common following cardiac surgery. J Cardiothorac Vasc Anaesth 5:201–208

Role of Blood Gas Measurements in the Management of Acute Asthma

D. Quoc Tuan

Introduction

Acute severe asthma is a frequent clinical condition which, despite modern therapies, continues to be associated with a high mortality rate. Intense bronchospasm leads to decreased alveolar ventilation which causes hypercapnia and alterations in blood pH as well as hypoxia. The use of blood gas measurements in the management of acute asthma is well documented in the literature, but so far they have been little used in Vietnam. The present study was designed to investigate changes in blood gas and acid–base balance in acute, severe asthma and to assess the role of these measurements in decisions relating to the use of mechanical ventilation in asthmatic patients.

Methods

The subjects of this study were 13 patients with severe asthma (mean age, 35 years; range, 17–65 years) who were admitted to the intensive care unit and who had no other complications. Blood gas analysis was performed during the asthma attack, which was usually on admission or soon afterwards. Further analyses were made one to three times per day during the therapeutic course and when the attack was over. Samples were collected from the radial artery and analysed on a JBA-7 blood gas analyser (Jookoo, Japan). Patients were treated with salbutamol and/or diaphylline and/or i.v. infusion of adrenaline, combined with oxygenation and i.v. corticosteroids. Mechanical ventilation was provided with an Acoma 100 ventilator.

Results

Results for $PaCO_2$ and pH during the attack are shown in Table 1. Table 2 shows a comparison of the values for $PaCO_2$, PaO_2 and pH during an attack and after treatment. The relationship between $PaCO_2$ and pH values following drug therapy and the need for mechanical ventilation is shown in Table 3.

Table 1. $PaCO_2$ and pH measurements during an acute asthma attack

Measurements	Patients (n)
$PaCO_2$ (mmHg)	
<45	0
45–50	3
>50	10
pH	
<7.20	4
7.20–7.30	3
7.30–7.35	4
>7.35	3

Table 2. Comparison of $PaCO_2$, PaO_2 and pH measurements during an acute asthma attack and after treatment

	During attack	After treatment	p value
$PaCO_2$	59.2±10.4	36.8±4.8	<0.01
PaO_2	95.4±30.0	83.0±6.2	>0.05
pH	7.25±0.17	7.42±0.02	<0.01

Table 3. $PaCO_2$ and pH values and mechanical ventilation (MV) in patients after drug therapy

	With MV (n)	Without (n)	Total (n)
$PaCO_2$ (mmHg)			
<50	0	3	3
>50	10	0	10
pH			
≥7.35	0	2	2
7.35–7.30	3	1	4
<7.30	7	0	7

Conclusions

We conclude from this study that normal or increased $PaCO_2$ is a common sign in acute severe asthma and that a $PaCO_2$ of over 50 mmHg after drug therapy is an important indicator for treatment with mechanical ventilation. Changes in $PaCO_2$ are reflected in decreased pH, and when this falls below 7.30 and is accompanied by clinical signs of disturbed breathing, mechanical ventilation should be the treatment of choice.

Relevance of End-Tidal Carbon Dioxide Monitoring in Ventilated Neonates

S. Nangia, A. Saili, and A.K. Dutta

Introduction

Arterial blood gases (ABG) are the gold standard for assessing the adequacy of ventilation, and all non-invasive monitoring methods should be correlated with ABG. The present study was undertaken to monitor end-tidal carbon dioxide in ventilated neonates to assess its reliability as a function of $PaCO_2$ and also to correlate it with $PaCO_2$ in different clinical situations.

Methods

End-tidal CO_2 monitoring was carried out prospectively in all ventilated neonates in a neonatal intensive care unit who were admitted from March to August 1995, irrespective of the birth weight and gestation of the baby or of any indication for ventilation. ABG were obtained in all ventilated babies together with simultaneous, continuous End-tidal CO_2 monitoring with a Datex Cardiocap and a paediatric End-tidal tube. The blood gas samples were analysed on an AVL 995 Hb blood gas analyser, and End-tidal CO_2 was analysed continuously by a side stream using a Datex Cardiocap II monitor.

Results

A total of 152 samples taken from in-dwelling radial artery catheters were analysed from babies with birth weights ranging from 900 to 3400 g (gestation age, 28–42 weeks) ventilated for various conditions, including severe birth asphyxia (SBA), meconium aspiration syndrome (MAS), recurrent apnoea (RA) and hyaline membrane disease (HMD).

Statistical analysis to determine whether there was a correlation between End-tidal CO_2 and its corresponding $PaCO_2$ value was carried out according to ten groups as follows: three groups for birth weight, <1.5 kg, 1.5–2.5 kg and >2.5 kg; three groups for gestational age, 28–31±6 weeks, 32–36±6 weeks, 37–41±6 weeks; four groups as determined by the need for ventilation in the various conditions.

The correlation coefficients in the ten groups ranged from 0.55 to 0.96, and the correlation between End-tidal CO_2 and $PaCO_2$ was highly significant ($p<0.01$) in the case of babies weighing more than 2.5 kg and in the group weighing 1.5–2.5 kg, in term and pre-term 32- to 36-week babies, and in babies with MAS, SBA and RA. The lowest correlation coefficient (0.55) was in babies with HMD.

Conclusions

This study showed that End-tidal CO_2 correlates closely with $PaCO_2$ in most clinical conditions in neonates, and it is recommended that End-tidal CO_2 be measured in ventilated babies in all level III neonatal intensive care units.

Trace Element Deficiency in Critically Ill Patients

A. Kogan, P. Singer, J. Cohen, Y. Broza, and O. Zinder

Introduction

Trace elements play a key role in homeostasis, but very little is known about the levels of trace elements in critically ill patients. The aim of this study was to evaluate plasma concentrations of two important trace elements, zinc and copper, in the initial 24 h after admission to the intensive care unit and to assess the relationship between these measurements and variables such as age, length of stay in the intensive care unit and the Acute Physiology and Chronic Health Evaluation (APACHE) II (severity) score.

Methods

Measurements were made on 20 consecutive patients who were being ventilated (nine medical, eight surgical and three multiple trauma patients). The measurements were as follows: zinc and copper, which were determined by atomic absorption spectrophotometry; magnesium, phosphate, calcium, albumin and blood urea nitrogen, which were determined by automated spectrophotometric analysis.

Results

The results of the various parameters are shown in Table 1. All the zinc levels (range, 2.3–14.2 µmol/l) and the majority of the copper levels (range, 6.3–33.4 µmol/l) were lower than the accepted reference ranges. There was no significant relationship between zinc or copper concentrations and age, APACHE score or length of stay in the intensive care unit. Zinc levels were correlated to copper levels (r, 0.49; $p<0.02$) and to albumin (r, 0.55; $p<0.01$), while copper levels were correlated to albumin (r, 0.44; $p<0.05$) and the zinc to copper ratio was correlated to blood urea nitrogen (BUN; r, 0.43; $p<0.05$).

Table 1. Levels of trace elements in patients being ventilated

Parameter	Mean±SD
Age (years)	61.5±17.6
APACHE II	9.8±6
Stay in ICU (days)	8.3±7.3
Mg (mmol/l)	0.94±0.20
Phosphate (mmol/l)	1.40±0.67
Ca (mmol/l)	2.09±0.15
BUN (mmol/l)	12.1±12.8
Albumin (g/l)	30±10
Zn (μmol/l)	7.64±3.82
Cu (μmol/l)	14.9±5.8
Zn/Cu ratio	0.54±0.29
Zn/albumin ratio	0.25±0.11

APACHE, Acute Physiology and Chronic Health Evaluation score; ICU, intensive care unit; BUN, blood urea nitrogen.

Conclusions

The fall in serum zinc concentrations in critically ill patients was greater than the fall in albumin concentrations. This may indicate an active transfer of zinc ions to another tissue compartment. The significant relationship between zinc and copper may indicate similar mechanisms in their metabolic pathways. The relationship between the zinc to copper ratio and BUN suggests a change due to specific disease states, e.g. renal failure. These findings may be useful in the assessment of zinc and copper requirements in critically ill patients.

Electrolyte and Acid–Base Balance in Respiratory and Metabolic Acidosis

V. Cosic, M. Rancic, and B. V. Dordevic

Introduction

The potential complexity of acid–base disorders sometimes makes it necessary to measure parameters other than merely pH and blood gases in order to make a diagnosis; the aim of this study was to evaluate the role of a range of biochemical and haematological tests in the evaluation of patients with respiratory or metabolic acidosis.

Methods

Measurements were performed in 36 patients with chronic obstructive pulmonary disease (COPD) and in 11 patients with diabetic ketoacidosis (DKA). These results were compared with a control group of 36 volunteers. The acid–base and electrolyte measurements were made on standard AVL blood gas and electrolyte analysers. Haematological measurements were made by standard laboratory methods, and lactate was measured by an ultraviolet (UV) spectrophotometric method.

Results

Tables 1 and 2 show the results of the various parameters in the control group and in the two groups of patients. The main features in the patients with COPD were a normal pH, significantly lower PaO_2 and oxygen saturation, but significantly increased $PaCO_2$ (hypercapnia) and bicarbonate; this corresponds to a compensated respiratory acidosis. By determining standard HCO_3, it was possible to calculate that the HCO_3 had increased 0.59 mmol/l for every 1 mmHg increase in $PaCO_2$. Such an increase in HCO_3 excluded the possibility of a mixed acid–base disorder. The COPD patients also had significantly higher haemoglobin concentration and alveolar to arterial difference for oxygen ($AaDO_2$), but values for alveolar to arterial oxygen partial pressure ratio (a/A) and oxygen content of arterial blood (CaO_2) were lower, thereby confirming the existence of hypoxaemia and serious disturbances in

Table 1. Acid–base parameters (mean±SE) in controls and patients with chronic obstructive pulmonary disease (COPD) or diabetic ketoacidosis (DKA)

Parameter	COPD patients	DKA patients	Controls
pH	7.385±0.003	7.076±0.067	7.402±0.002
$PaCO_2$ (mmHg)	64.95±1.38	26.20±2.85	40.21±0.86
PaO_2 (mmHg)	37.52±1.05		88.2±1.24
HCO_3 (mmol/l)	38.61±10.87	8.12±1.96	24.3±0.6
BE (mmol/l)	10.57±0.69	−19.06±2.41	−1.01±0.26
SaO_2 (1/1)	0.67±0.02		0.97±0.02
$AaDO_2$ (mmHg)	28.32±0.81		8.31±0.21
a/A	0.57±0.04		0.91±0.04
CaO_2 (ml/l)	146.1±0.3		181.0±10.0

BE, base excess; SaO_2, arterial oxygen saturation; $AaDO_2$, alveolar to arterial difference for oxygen; a/A, alveolar to arterial oxygen partial pressure.

Table 2. Haematological, electrolyte and lactate values (mean±SE) in controls and patients with chronic obstructive pulmonary disease (COPD) or diabetic ketoacidosis (DKA)

Parameter	COPD patients	DKA patients	Controls
Haemoglobin (g/l)	156.0±8.6		132.3±7.6
Haematocrit (1/1)	0.58±0.01	0.37±0.05	0.46±0.05
Na (mmol/l)	141.8±0.49	136.6±0.56	136.6±0.3
K (mmol/l)	6.23±0.12	4.11±0.28	4.68±0.11
Erythrocyte K (mmol/l)	99.15±1.31	96.3±2.9	101.0±1.15
Cl (mmol/l)	92.31±10.96	98.3±3.9	101.0±0.45
Ca^{2+} (mmol/l)	1.32±0.07		1.20±0.05
Mg (mmol/l)	0.88±0.08		1.01±0.07
Lactate (mmol/l)	3.84±0.14		1.86±0.11

ventilation. Hypoxaemia was also the cause of the significantly elevated lactate level, while the acidosis was the cause of the hyperkalaemia.

In contrast, the patients with DKA had a significant metabolic acidosis with decreased values of pH, $PaCO_2$ and HCO_3. By using standard pH, the decrease in $PaCO_2$, resulting from hyperventilation, was shown to cause an increase in pH of 0.148 and represented some degree of compensation for the loss of bicarbonate. The increased anion gap in these patients was due to the presence of organic anions, hydroxybutyrate, acetoacetate and lactate and explains the reduction in bicarbonate. The decreased serum potassium is characteristic of potassium depletion early in DKA, which is confirmed by a lower erythrocyte potassium level.

Conclusions

We conclude that it is necessary to determine all of the above-mentioned parameters and those shown in Tables 1 and 2 in order for a correct evaluation of primary acidosis to be made, for the existence of mixed disorders to be determined and for the extent of any compensatory response to be measured.

Point-of-Care Testing of Haemoglobin Derivatives by Co-Oximetry with Simultaneous Blood Gas Measurements

M. L. S. Fong, and I. K. Tan

Introduction

The blood gas analyser has recently become a vital part of critical care management and is mandatory in most intensive care units. However, blood gas results alone can sometimes be misleading in the presence of dyshaemoglobinaemia. Recent advances in technology have made it possible for measurements of blood gases and haemoglobin derivatives to be interfaced as one unit or combined within the same instrument. We have evaluated the performance of two such co-oximetry instruments.

Methods

The Radiometer ABL 520 pH/blood gas analyser incorporates a co-oximeter which, after ultrasonic haemolysis of the blood, measures oxyhaemoglobin, reduced haemoglobin, methaemoglobin (MetHb) and carboxyhaemoglobin (COHb) by spectrophotometry. The AVL 912 Co-oxylite can be interfaced to a blood gas analyser, has measurement principles similar to the Radiometer instrument and measures the same parameters plus sulphhaemoglobin (SHb). The instruments were evaluated for linearity, precision and agreement with standard methods and between the two instruments. Varying concentrations of COHb were produced by bubbling commercial methane gas into whole blood, and for MetHb an excess of sodium nitrite was added to whole blood.

Results

The precision of the two instruments at varying concentrations of COHb, MetHb and SHb is shown in Tables 1 and 2. The linearity of the COHb and MetHb methods and the correlation of the total haemoglobin determination with the Technicon H1 method is shown in Table 3. The correlation between the Radiometer and AVL instruments was 0.9905 for COHb and 0.9906 for MetHb.

Table 1. Precision of the Radiometer ABL 520 at varying concentrations of carboxyhaemoglobin (COHb), methaemoglobin (MetHb) and sulphhaemoglobin (SHb)

	COHb			MetHb			SHb		
Level (%)	0.76	5.20	51.52	0.58	5.05	50.59	–	–	–
CV%	16.6	2.2	2.7	35.2	4.2	0.8	–	–	–

Table 2. Precision of the AVL 912 at varying concentrations of carboxyhaemoglobin (COHb), methaemoglobin (MetHb) and sulphhaemoglobin (SHb)

	COHb			MetHb			SHb		
Level (%)	0.99	4.74	50.05	0.56	4.15	44.78	0.5	1.3	1.9
CV%	11.1	3.7	0.9	13.6	5.0	1.2	0.0	0.0	0.0

Table 3. Linearity of the carboxyhaemoglobin (COHb) and methaemoglobin (MetHb) methods and correlation of total haemoglobin determination with the Technicon H1 method

	Radiometer 520	AVL 912
Limit of COHB linearity (%)	96	99.8
Limit of MetHb linearity (%)	96	80
THb correlation with Technicon H1 method	0.9991	0.9975

Conclusions

The performance of both these instruments was satisfactory. The major advantage of co-oximetry instruments is that, as well as quantifying abnormal concentrations of the various haemoglobins, they also provide a more accurate determination of oxygen saturation in the presence of dyshaemoglobinaemia.

Changes in Body Water Compartments in Children with Meningitis

V. Kumar, P. Singhi, and S. Singhi

Introduction

The fluid requirement in critically ill children with meningitis is influenced by the body water changes occurring in response to the illness, and whether to restrict fluids as a routine therapeutic measure has been a matter of continuing debate. The aim of this study was to provide data to clarify this issue by evaluating the changes in body water and electrolytes in children with acute meningitis to examine their relationship with severity and patient outcome.

Methods

The subjects in this study were 30 children (age range, 2 months to 5 years) with acute meningitis and 30 age- and sex-matched controls. Total body water (TBW), extracellular water (ECW), and serum and urinary sodium (Na) were measured on day 1 and after recovery.

Results

The TBW and ECW results in the patients and controls are shown in Table 1. The mean ECW excess was 33 ml/kg, with the excess being 70±8 ml/kg in the severely ill, 50±32 ml/kg in the moderately ill and 12±18 ml/kg in mildly ill children ($p<0.01$). Those who had complications had much higher ECW (49 ml/kg) than those who recovered completely (17±27 ml/kg). The only significant determinant of ECW excess was severity of illness (partial r^2, 0.62). The syndrome of inappropriate antidiuretic hormone (ADH) secretion (SIADH) was diagnosed in 14 children, each having an ECW excess of more than 45 ml/kg. There was a significant inverse correlation between serum sodium and excess ECW (r, –0.82).

Table 1. Total body water (TBW) and extracellular water (ECW) in patients and controls (mean±SD)

		Patients	
	Controls	Day 1	Recovery
TBW (ml/kg)	642±49	683±63*	643±48
EBW (ml/kg)	271±62	311±76*	271±63

* $p > 0.05$ vs. controls

Conclusions

Only those children with meningitis who have SIADH need fluid restriction. The severity of the illness and the serum sodium can be used as a guide for therapy.

Surfactant as a Marker of Disease Severity in Critically Ill Patients with Respiratory Failure

I. Doyle and A. D. Bersten

Introduction

Alveolar surfactant is fundamental for normal lung function. We recently reported increased concentrations of surfactant protein A (SP-A) in serum from patients with acute respiratory failure (ARF). Since surfactant protein B (SP-B) is synthesised as a precursor (approximately 42 kDa) considerably smaller than alveolar (A) SP-A (approximately 650 kDa) and since little is known about surfactant status in patients with ARF, the aims of this study were to determine whether SP-B enters the circulation more readily than SP-A and to examine surfactant composition in the injured lung.

Methods

Blood was collected from normal individuals (controls) and from ventilated patients with either no evidence of cardiorespiratory disease (OD), acute cardiogenic pulmonary oedema (APE) or acute respiratory distress syndrome (ARDS). Surfactant composition in tracheal aspirate fluid (ASP) was examined in a separate cohort of patients, either with, or at risk of, ARDS. SP-A and B were measured by enzyme-linked immunosorbent assay (ELISA). ASP phospholipids and disaturated phospholipids (DSP) were measured and phospholipid classes quantified by high-performance liquid chromatography (HPLC). All analyses were performed in a randomised, blind manner.

Results

Plasma SP-A and SP-B levels at enrolment are shown in Table 1. Plasma SP-A and SP-B levels were elevated in the APE and ARDS patients relative to the controls and OD patients ($p<0.001$ in all comparisons, Mann-Whitney test). During the course of their admission, plasma SP-A and SP-B were inversely related to blood oxygenation (PaO_2/FiO_2; $p<0.0001$, $n=260$; Spearman) and static respiratory system compliance ($\Delta V/\Delta P$; $p<0.0001$, $n=168$). Plasma SP-B/SP-A was also inversely related to PaO_2/FiO_2 ($p<0.026$) and $\Delta V/\Delta P$

Table 1. Plasma surfactant protein A (SP-A) and SP-B levels at enrolment (mean±SE)

Plasma	Controls ($n=33$)	OD ($n=7$)	APE ($n=10$)	ARDS ($n=22$)
SP-A (ng/ml)	17±37	177±16	264±22	478±58
SP-B (ng/ml)	1685±58	1829±635	3646±635	8007±1654

OD, patients with no evidence of cardiorespiratory disease; APE, patients with acute cardiogenic pulmonary oedema; ARDS, patients with acute respiratory distress syndrome.

Table 2. Correlations

	PaO_2/FiO_2	Eprv-st	Ers-dyn	$\%E_2$
Alv SP-A	0.73*	0.55**	−0.06	−0.65*
Alv SP-B	0.74*	0.60**	−0.06	−0.54**
DSP	0.67*	0.56**	−0.21	−0.73*
PC	0.65*	0.61**	0.03	−0.67*
SPH/PL	−0.64*	−0.54**	−0.06	0.64*

Eprv-st, static elastance of the positive end-expiratory pressure (PEEP)-recruited volume; Ers-dyn, dynamic respiratory elastance; $\%E_2$, volume-dependent component of Ers-dyn; SP, surfactant protein; DSP, disaturated phospholipids; PC, phosphatidylcholine; SPH, sphingomyelin.

* $p<0.01$; ** $p<0.05$.

($p<0.009$). Individually, daily changes in lung function were acutely reflected in concomitant variations in plasma SP-A, SP-B and SP-B/SP-A.

When normalised to sphingomyelin (SPH), alveolar SP-A and SP-B, DSP and phosphatidylcholine (PC) correlated directly with PaO_2/FiO_2 and static elastance of the positive end-expiratory pressure (PEEP)-recruited volume (Eprv-st), whereas SPH/PL was inversely related to both. When dynamic respiratory elastance (Ers-dyn; 1/compliance) and its volume-dependent component ($\%E_2$), representing lung hyperinflation, were determined; alveolar SP-A and SP-B, DSP and PC were inversely related to $\%E_2$, whereas SPH/PL was directly related. The correlation values for these various relationships are shown in Table 2.

Conclusions

We concluded that SP-B enters the circulation more readily than SP-A in a manner reflecting the severity of lung injury and that surfactant deficiency is a major factor contributing to hypoxaemia and lung hyperinflation in ARF.

Reliability of the Pulse Oximeter

B.G. Lee, P.T. Morley, and J.F. Cade

Introduction

Despite the fact that pulse oximeters are now used routinely in most intensive care units, clinical experience suggests that the results from these non-invasive instruments do not always correlate with results for oxygen saturation from conventional blood gas analysis. The aim of this study was to directly compare the results obtained by pulse oximetry to those obtained by a blood gas analyser and co-oximeter.

Methods

A total of 100 patient samples with varying levels of perfusion, haemoglobin, oxygenation and temperature were analysed in the study. Four commonly used pulse oximeters were compared: Nellcor N200, Nellcor N100, Ohmeda Biox 3700 and Criticare 501+. The instruments were attached to the patient and allowed to stabilise and then results from the instrument were recorded. Simultaneously, arterial samples were collected for blood gas and co-oximetry measurements using a Radiometer ABL3, which provides a calculated saturation, and a Radiometer OSM3, which provides the most accurate measurement of oxygen saturation.

Results

The correlation between the saturations obtained by each of the oximeters, the calculated saturation obtained from the ABL3 blood gas instrument and the saturation obtained by the OSM3 is shown in Table 1. Also shown is the approximate correction factor that would convert the measured saturations to that achieved by the OSM3 instrument.

There was a high degree of correlation between all the instruments and the OSM3 co-oximeter. However, systematic differences existed between the instruments, presumably due to differences in the algorithms used to calculate saturation.

Table 1. Correlation between saturations and approximate correction factor

	Nellcor N200	Nellcor N100	Ohmeda 3700	Critcare 501+	ABL3
Correlation	0.95	0.94	0.92	0.94	0.91
Correction	0	0	+2.5	+1.5	+2

Conclusions

Our results confirm that, in most situations, pulse oximeters provide a satisfactory estimate of oxygen saturation; in fact, two instruments provided more accurate answers than the blood gas analyser. Proper use of pulse oximeters, which includes awareness of any systematic differences that the device has from the absolute standard, should diminish the requirement for confirmatory blood gas analysis.

Nephrology

Evidence of Oxidant Injury in Patients with Post-Diarrhoeal Acute Renal Failure

S. Rao, K. V. Murty, K. S. Saibaba, S. Somaiah, and M. V. Bhaskar

Introduction

Previous animal studies have demonstrated oxidant injury in both toxic and ischaemic acute renal failure. The aim of this study was to look for evidence of oxidant injury and alterations in thyroid hormones in acute renal failure as a complication of diarrhoeal disease, a common condition in India.

Methods

Measurements were made in ten patients with post-diarrhoeal acute renal failure and in 15 healthy volunteers as control subjects. Indications of oxidant injury were determined from measurements of lipid peroxides (LPO), superoxide dismutase (SOD) and glutathione peroxidase (GPO). Other parameters which were measured included plasma iron and ferritin, while thyroid status was assessed by measuring total tri-iodothyronine (T_3), total thyroxin (T_4) and free T_4.

Results

A comparison between patient and control results obtained on admission for oxidant and iron status is shown in Table 1. With the exception of GPO, the increase in all parameters on admission persisted at 1 week, although LPO and SOD had started to decline. The decline in GPO was only statistically significant after 1 week.

Table 2 shows the results for thyroid status. Only total T3 showed an increase towards normal levels after 1 week of hospitalisation. None of the thyroid function tests correlated with plasma LPO levels.

Table 1. Oxidant and iron status on admission of patients and controls (mean±SD)

	LPO (nmol/ml)	SOD (U/ml)	GPO (U/l)		Iron (µg/dl)
			On admission	After 1 week	
Patients	2.50±0.5	0.27±0.27	446±199	302±178	200±8
Controls	1.03±0.58	0.05±0.02	540±98	540±98	110±18
p value	p<0.001	p<0.05	NS	p<0.001	p<0.01

LPO, lipid peroxides; SOD, superoxide dismutase; GOP, glutathione peroxidase; NS, not significant.

Table 2. Thyroid status

	Total T_3 (nmol/l)	Total T_4 (nmol/l)	Free T_4 (pmol/l)
Patients	1.2±0.5	54±24	10.3±7.1
Controls	1.9±0.5	88±27	16.3±.4
p value	p<0.001	p<0.01	p<0.01

T_3, Tri-iodothyronine; T_4, thyroxine.

Conclusions

The data from this study suggest that reactive oxygen species may be involved in post-diarrhoeal acute renal failure, but that thyroid hormones are unlikely to be involved in oxidant injury.

Gastroenterology

Sensitivity and Specificity of Different Plasma Enzyme Assays in the Diagnosis of Acute Pancreatitis

S. Ignjatovic, M. Todorovic, M. Gvozdenovic, and D. Mirkovic

Introduction

The differential diagnosis of acute pancreatitits can be difficult. Although clinical history and physical examination are helpful, measurement of serum enzyme levels is an important part of the evaluation of patients with acute abdominal pain and possible pancreatitis. The aim of this study was to evaluate the usefulness of measurement for lipase (EC 3.1.1.3), pancreatic iso-amylase and amylase (EC 3.2.1.1) in the differential diagnosis of pancreatitis.

Methods

Lipase was assayed (with colipase) by a turbidometric method, pancreatic iso-amylase by double monoclonal antibody (immunoinhibition) technique and amylase by paranitrophenol glycoside-7 ethylidine-blocked substrate. We investigated 38 patients with acute pancreatitis (25 men, 13 women; age range, 21–64 years) and 81 patients with gastrointestinal disease of extrapancreatic origin (44 men, 37 women; age range, 21–64 years). The following diagnoses were made in the latter group of patients: acute appendicitis ($n=42$), exacerbated peptic ulcer ($n=11$), bilary colic ($n=8$) and peritonitis ($n=20$). The diagnosis was based on clinical assessment in conjunction with laboratory and radiological procedures, including ultrasound and computed tomography. The diagnostic sensitivity and specificity of the enzyme analyses were assessed using receiver operator curve (ROC) analysis with calculation of ROC curves, area under the curve (AUC) and standard errors by GraphRoc software.

Results

The technical performance of all three assays was satisfactory, with within-run precision or coefficient of variation (CV) ranging from 0.4% to 4.8% and between run CV ranging from 0.9% to 6.9%. The enzyme activities on admission for pancreatitis-positive and pancreatitis-negative patients are shown in Table 1.

Table 1. Enzyme activities in pancreatitis-positive and -negative patients on admission

| Group | Patients (*n*) | Lipase (U/l) | | Isoamylase (U/l) | | Amylase (U/l) |
		Mean±SD	Range	Mean±SD	Range	Mean±SD
Pancreatitis positive	38	1598±1242	215–5766	614±418	24–1680	824±577
Pancreatitis negative	81	151±137	28–750	29±39	3–210	69±64

Table 2. Receiver operator curve (ROC) analysis of enzymes (mean±SE)

	Lipase	Isoamylase	Amylase
ROC AUC[a]	0.9903±0.0082	0.9829±0.0088	0.9717±0.0125
Cut-off value (U/l)	573	131	213
Diagnostic efficiency	0.94	0.93	0.89

[a] AUC, area under curve.

ROC analysis, including computation of the ROC AUC, showed that the best classification of patients came from lipase and pancreatic isoamylase, as shown by the results given in Table 2.

Conclusions

This study has confirmed the diagnostic value of plasma lipase and pancreatic isoamylase assays. The value of amylase as an additional test for the diagnosis of acute pancreatitis can be improved by using a cut-off value of approximately three times the upper limit of the reference range.

Urinary Trypsinogen-2 Test Strip –
A New Rapid Test for Acute Pancreatitis

J. Hedstrom, A. Korvuo, P. Kenkimaki, S. Tikanoja,
R. Haapiaainen, E. Kivilaakso, and U. Stenman

Introduction

Early diagnosis of acute pancreatitis (AP) is important, as serious complications such as fulminant organ system failure and pancreatic necrosis or sepsis occur in 20%–30% of cases. Furthermore, intensive therapy of severe AP is more likely to be effective if it can be instituted at an early stage. However, the clinical features of AP can be atypical or hard to distinguish from other acute abdominal conditions, and the diagnosis may be overlooked at the initial examination. Therefore, there is a considerable need for a rapid and reliable test which can differentiate between AP and other abdominal conditions at an early stage. Earlier studies have suggested that there is a relationship between serum levels of the proteolytic enzyme trypsinogen-2 and pancreatic damage [1], while more recent work has demonstrated increased urine and serum levels of trypinogen-2 in AP [2]. Based on promising results with a quantitative test for trypsinogen-2 in urine, which is markedly increased in patients with AP, we have developed a rapid test strip for detection of trypsinogen-2 in urine and evaluated its utility in the diagnosis of AP.

Methods

The measurement principle of the test strip relies on immunochromatography utilising two monoclonal antibodies specific for two different epitopes on the trypsinogen-2 molecule. One antibody is immobilised onto a nitrocellulose membrane, and the other onto blue latex particles The test is carried out by dipping the strip into urine so that all the trypsinogen-2 in the sample binds to the antibody-labelled latex particles, which then migrate with the sample fluid across the nitrocellulose membrane into a catching zone containing the second antibody.

Results

A trypsinogen-2 concentration of more than 50 µg/l in the sample resulted in a blue line in the catching zone within 3 min. The clinical utility of the method was tested on urine samples from 57 patients with AP, 40 patients with acute abdominal extrapancreatic disease and 57 patients without evidence of abdominal disease. From the results obtained on these samples, the sensitivity was 91% and specificity was 90% in differentiating AP from acute abdominal extrapancreatic disease. The rapid strip test gave results similar to the quantitative assay in 98% of cases.

Conclusions

Our results show that the trypsinogen-2 test strip has a high accuracy for the diagnosis of AP. The test is rapid and easy to perform and therefore may become a useful tool in screening patients for suspected AP in doctor's offices and out-patient departments which lack access to laboratory facilities.

References

1. Itkonen O, Koivunen E, Hurme M et al (1990) Time-resolved immunofluorometric assays for trypsinogen-1 and -2 in serum reveal preferential elevation of trypsinogen-2 in pancreatitis. J Lab Clin Med 115:712–718
2. Hedstrom J, Leinonen J, Sainio V et al (1994) Time-resolved immunofluorometric assays for trypsin-2 complexed with alpha-1-antitrypsin in serum. Clin Chem 40:1761–1765

Gastrointestinal Mucosal Permeability in Critically Ill Patients

A. E. Rodriguez, R. Conejero, M. Planes, J. Acosta,
A. Bonet, J. Lopez, R. Nunez, and A. Mesajo

Introduction

The gut mucosa usually operates as a barrier limiting the systemic absorption of luminal microbes. Under certain conditions, namely sepsis, circulatory shock, intestinal paralysis, bacterial overgrowth and absence of enteral nutrition, the intestinal mucosa is unable to perform this barrier function. This loss of function may be a contributing factor in the development of multiple organ failure. Although bacterial translocation in humans after injury has not been demonstrated, a number of studies suggest that there is substantial disruption of the barrier function of the gut in critically ill patients. Gut mucosal permeability can be assessed by the ratio of small-molecule to large-molecule permeability. The objectives of the study were to measure the gut permeability in critically ill patients using a dual sugar test and to assess these measurements in relation to patient outcome.

Methods

The subjects in the study were 54 critically ill patients and 14 healthy volunteers to act as controls. Gut permeability was assessed from measurements of lactulose and mannitol in urine using enzymatic methods after loading doses of the two sugars; the percentage recoveries of lactulose and mannitol were expressed as a ratio [1]. These measurements were carried out at baseline and at days 3 and 5.

Results

There was a significant increase in the lactulose to mannitol excretion ratio in the patients at days 0, 3 and 5 (0.28, 0.26 and 0.20, respectively) as compared to the controls ($p=0.03$). The increase was related to the Acute Physiology and Chronic Health Evaluation (APACHE) II severity score and was more marked in those patients who developed sepsis and in those who developed infections in the intensive care unit.

Conclusions

Our results suggest that atrophy of the gastrointestinal mucosa with inadequate gut barrier function may develop in critically ill patients. These alterations may be particularly significant in those patients who develop sepsis. Since gastrointestinal permeability plays a major role in the metabolic response after injury, these findings may be of clinical relevance to the daily management of critically ill patients.

References

1. Northrop CA, Lunn PG, Behrens RH (1990) Automated enzymatic assays for the determination of intestinal permeability probes in urine. 1. Lactulose and lactose. Clin Chim Acta 187:79–88

Haematology – Haemostasis

Altered Coagulability in Ischaemic Heart Disease

A. Rizk, S. Mokhtar, A.S. El-Deen, S. Nguib, and M. El-Ansary

Introduction

Clinical interest in coronary artery disease has previously concentrated on the pathological changes in lipid metabolism and their effects upon the structure of the arterial wall. More recently, the focus has moved to studies of altered coagulability, and the aim of this study was to identify which patients with coronary heart disease have abnormal coagulation parameters.

Methods

The subjects of this study were 66 patients with coronary heart disease who were divided into three groups: 26 patients with acute myocardial infarction (MI), 20 patients with a previous MI and 20 patients with unstable angina but no previous MI. All patients had normal liver and renal function tests. In addition, there were 30 control subjects. Plasma samples were withdrawn from all patients following their admission to the critical care department and were analysed for procoagulants, i.e. β-thromboglobulin (BTG), factor VIII C activity and kallikrein, and for anticoagulants, i.e. protein C activity and fibrinolytic marker fibrin degradation products (FDP).

Results

The results of the various parameters in the patients and control groups are shown in Table 1. Compared to the control group, the three patient groups showed significantly higher levels of the procoagulants BTG, factor VIII C and kallikrein. The values for FDP were not significantly different, but both groups with MI had significantly lower values for protein C.

Table 1. Procoagulants and anticoagulants in patients with acute myocardial infarction (MI), with previous MI, with unstable angina and in controls (mean±SD)

Group C (%[a])	BTG (IU/ml)	Factor VIII C (%[a])	Kallikrein (IU/ml)	Protein	FDP (μg/ml)
Controls	29±9	152±32	2±0.7	81±6.6	2.9±1.1
Acute MI	203±49	254±90	2.3±0.3	66±21	2.7±1.2
Previous MI	397±140	253±110	2.6±0.3	70±17	3.2±1.5
Angina	292±86	192±66	2.6±0.5	83±17	3.1±1.3

BTG, β-Thromboglobulin; FDP, fibrin degradation products.
[a] Percentage of normal.

Conclusions

The procoagulants BTG, factor VIII C and kallikrein reflect a tendency towards developing thrombosis rather than indicating recent thrombosis, and abnormal results may therefore be of prognostic rather than diagnostic value. The significant decrease in protein C correspondingly reflects a decreased tendency towards anticoagulation and is therefore an indirect marker for a hypercoagulable state. Routine measurements of procoagulants and anticoagulants in patients with ischaemic heart disease may serve to identify patients with a hypercoagulable state and to identify subjects susceptible to events so that appropriate therapy may be provided.

Plasminogen Activator Inhibitor in Acute Myocardial Infarction: A Predictor of Spontaneous Lysis and Patency of Infarct-Related Artery

A. El-Naggar, A. Rizk, S. El-Tobgy, and S. Mokhtar

Introduction

It is now widely accepted that thrombosis is one mechanism – and perhaps the most important one – in acute myocardial infarction. As a result of this knowledge, thrombolytic therapy has gained widespread acceptance. However, there is considerable debate about the relative importance of spontaneous lysis versus drug-induced thrombolysis. Accordingly, the aim of this study was to assess the relationship between the fibrinolytic system and successful reperfusion in patients with myocardial infarction.

Methods

The study was carried out on 70 patients who had suffered a myocardial infarction (63 males, seven females; mean age, 52 years) and 35 age-matched control subjects. As an index of the fibrinolytic system, plasminogen activator inhibitor (PAI) was measured before treatment, 3 h after treatment and then on days 3, 5 and 7 after treatment. Treatment consisted of either i.v. nitroglycerine or streptokinase. Coronary angiography was performed on all patients within 7 days of admission.

Results

Of the 32 patients who received nitroglycerine, ten (28%) had patent infarct-related arteries on angiography, compared to 28 (71.8%) of the 38 patients treated with streptokinase ($p<0.001$). Results of PAI in the various groups are shown in Table 1. Serial measurements after treatment showed a subsequent decline in all PAI levels, but patients with occluded arteries had a slower decline and higher levels at any one time than those in patients with patent arteries (77 ± 48 vs. 48 ± 21, $p<0.03$).

Table 1. Plasminogen activator inhibitor (PAI) results in patients after treatment with nitroglycerine or streptokinase (ng/ml; mean±SD)

	Total	Nitroglycerine		Streptokinase	
		Occluded	Patent	Occluded	Patent
Controls	40±12				
Pretreatment	126±54*	175±49	86±78**	158±42	93±28***

* $p<0.0001$ vs. controls; ** $p<0.001$ vs. occluded group; *** $p<0.002$ vs. occluded group.

Conclusions

The data from this study shows that PAI may play an important role in myocardial infarction, with high levels interfering with natural fibrinolysis and defeating streptokinase-induced thrombolysis, while low levels may tend to favour patency of the infarct-related artery and may allow spontaneous lysis.

Rapid Detection of Plasma Glycocalicin
by a Latex Agglutination Test and Its Use
in the Differential Diagnosis of Thrombocytopaenia

S. Kunishima, S. Kobayashi, H. Saito, and T. Naoe

Introduction

The platelet membrane glycoprotein (GP) lb/IX complex plays a pivotal role in primary haemostasis, serving as a platelet receptor for von Willebrand factor. This complex contains three polypeptide chains: GPlb-α, GPlb-β and GPl-X. Glycocalicin is a soluble proteolytic fragment of GPlb-α and is normally present in the circulation. Previous work using an enzyme-linked immunosorbent assay has shown injury or platelet destruction in vivo [1]. The aim of this study was to develop a rapid assay for glycocalicin which could be used in the differential diagnosis of thrombocytopaenia.

Methods

Plasma glycocalicin was initially measured using a rapid latex agglutination technique [2]. Measurements were carried out on plasma from 36 control subjects and from 26 patients with thrombocytopaenia due to three different causes: idiopathic thrombocytopenia purpura (ITP, $n = 12$), aplastic anaemia (AA, $n = 4$) and myelodysplastic syndrome (MDS, $n = 10$).

Results

The results from the enzyme-linked immunosorbent assay showed normal levels of glycocalicin in plasma from ITP patients, where platelets are destroyed by immunological mechanisms, whereas markedly decreased levels of glycocalicin were present in the plasma of AA and MDS patients, where there is deficient platelet production. Furthermore, there was no overlap in the results between the ITP patients and those with AA or MDS. Results of the rapid latex agglutination assay on the plasma from the same patients are shown in Table 1. Plasma samples from all patients with ITP were positive in the assay, while all plasma from AA and MDS patients failed to agglutinate the latex.

Table 1. Results of the rapid latex agglutination assay (mean±SD) on plasma from idiopathic thrombocytopaenia purpura (ITP), aplastic anaemia (AA) and myelodysplastic syndrome (MDS) patients

Group	Subjects (n)	Concentration (μg/ml)	Titre
Controls	36	1.40±0.25	1–3
ITP	12	1.64±0.76	1–4
AA	4	0.08±0.02	0
MDS	10	0.19±0.15	0

Conclusions

The latex agglutination assay for plasma glycocalicin allows rapid discrimination of thrombocytopaenia due to impaired platelet production from that caused by increased platelet destruction. This method requires no special equipment and thus may be suitable for use as a screening test in point-of-care testing settings as well as in the routine clinical laboratory.

References

1. Kunishima S, Hayashi K, Kobayashi S et al (1991) New enzyme-linked immunosorbent assay for glycocalcin in plasma. Clin Chem 37:169–172
2. Kunishima S, Kobayashi S, Takagi A et al (1993) Rapid detection of plasma glycocalcin by a latex agglutination test. Am J Clin Pathol 100:579–582

New Technology

Monitoring of Multiple Pathophysiological Parameters in the Severely Head-Injured Patient

P. J. Kirkpatrick

Abstract

The continuous and simultaneous monitoring of different parameters in disease states of the brain has recently become available. They include measurements of intracranial pressure (ICP), cerebral perfusion pressure (CCP), jugular vein oxygen saturation (SjO_2), and cortical electrical activity. More recently, additional modalities have been introduced, such as transcranial Doppler (TCD), laser Doppler flowmeter (LDF) and near infrared spectroscopy (NIRS). In conjunction with computer support, these individual measurements can be combined into a multimodality computerised monitoring system, which may overcome the disadvantages of single procedures and provide more diagnostic power.

The aim of this study was to assess whether long-term monitoring with simultaneous registration using these newer modalities can provide information regarding the relative pathophysiological state of the brain in cerebral trauma, during and after therapy, on a day-to-day basis. Over a 24-month period, 104 severely head-injured patients were considered suitable for multimodality monitoring of the aforementioned parameters. In addition, 14 patients were monitored while receiving a mannitol infusion in order to determine whether real-time monitoring can also be employed to demonstrate the short-term pathophysiological response to a therapeutic manoeuvre.

Complete multimodality monitoring was successfully achieved in 24 patients with head trauma. Overall, 58 cerebral events were identified retrospectively in 16 patients. NIRS demonstrated changes in oxy- and deoxyhaemoglobin in approximately twice as many events as registered by jugular vein saturation measurements. In most patients, changes in cortical perfusion measured with LDF were tightly coupled to alterations in middle cerebral artery flow velocity (FV). Following mannitol infusion, the multimodality techniques demonstrated a rise in relative cerebral blood flow (CBF) which did not occur after isotonic saline.

Initial experience with bedside multimodality monitoring has been encouraging. It does appear possible to apply this procedure throughout the period of ventilation with a global signal reliability of approximately 50%. In addition, long-term monitoring using LDF provides information regarding the relative pathophysiological state of the brain as a consequence of brain oedema and increased ICP before, during and after different therapies on a day-to-day basis. Attempts to assess these patients have led us to consider the problem with a greater pathophysiological understanding in each individual case, allowing a more informed response and targeted therapy.

Introduction

The pathophysiological mechanisms excited after cerebral trauma are complex, but the contribution from brain ischaemia is recognised [76]. Ischaemic insults may continue after the primary cerebral insult, some of which could be avoidable [9, 49, 51]. Although the mechanisms causing brain injury are diverse, they operate to cause common pathophysiological changes, such as periods of raised ICP, derangements in CBF and brain hypoxia [10, 13, 64, 71]. The correct interpretation of such manifestations may ultimately assist in the clinical detection of brain ischaemia.

Changes in the pathophysiological state of the cerebral tissues may be transient, often lasting only a few minutes [34, 76]. Detection of such cerebral "events" has proved time-consuming and expensive. The technology requires considerable expert supervision and sophisticated computing and is therefore not yet suitable for routine clinical use. However, a recent impetus for continuing development has come from Robertson and colleagues who, using SjO_2 catheters, report that multiple episodes of brain hypoxia can be detected, which are associated with a poor clinical outcome [30, 71, 72]. Their efforts provide clear evidence supporting the clinical relevance of secondary cerebral events, implying that their detection and correction may be of some benefit.

Until recently, information on the condition of the brain after injury has depended largely upon imaging methods such as enhanced computed (CT) and emission tomography (ET). Intermittent monitoring with serial cranial imaging methods provides good spatial information, but cannot be repeated frequently enough to direct a clinical response [9, 29, 50, 63, 65]. In addition, the necessary intensive support for these patients is difficult to maintain within such imaging facilities. Thus methods for assessing brain function in an uninterrupted fashion have attracted increased clinical attention, particularly those that can be adapted for bedside monitoring, which reduces the need for patients transfer [10, 12, 15, 16, 43, 46, 48, 53, 73].

Interpretation of information gathered from cerebral monitors is of key importance in the future implementation of therapy. A single monitored cerebral event, such as a period of raised ICP, may be a manifestation of a variety of different pathophysiological changes. Cerebral swelling from ischaemia (oligaemia) and increased cerebral blood volume from hyperaemia are examples where the contrast in pathology is extreme. Blind ICP treatment in both instances using traditional dehydrating agents (such as mannitol) [86] may be beneficial in the former case, but may potentially aggravate the raised ICP in the latter. Directing therapy according to one measured parameter may therefore be inappropriate. Similarly, whereas controlled hyperventilation has traditionally been used to treat raised ICP by encouraging reactive vasoconstriction, recent evidence suggests that in situations of cerebral oligaemia these manoeuvres can increase cerebral ischaemia and lactate acid production. By monitoring several different parameters, each providing relevant information on different aspects of brain physiology, a greater understanding of the individual situation can be gathered. The aim would be to allow a more accurate targeting and policing of therapy. Computer support of multimodality monitoring is essential [14], helping the observer to identify important cerebral events from among the background noise and artefacts (frequently induced within the hostile environment of an intensive care unit), and provides assistance in the interpretation of complex information.

Continuous monitoring of different parameters concerning the health of the brain has recently become available. They include measurements of ICP, CPP, SjO_2 and cortical electrical activity [10, 12, 71, 72]. General systems monitors, such as pulse oximetry, end-tidal CO_2 and temperature are also clearly of importance. More recently, additional methods have been introduced, such as TCD [1, 15, 16, 32], LDF [46, 56, 57] and NIRS [31, 47]. Most of these methods have been employed in isolation and by themselves are open to different interpretation. Distinction from artefact can be difficult or impossible. It has therefore been my objective to monitor multiple variables to develop a multimodality computerised monitoring system which provides us with increased power for interpretation. Over the past 3 years we have developed such a service in the Neurointensive Care Unit in Addenbrookes Hospital, Cambridge (United Kingdom). The data presented concerns diffuse head injured patients, although more lately we have applied the methods to other coma-producing conditions.

The modalities that we now employ are ICP and arterial blood pressure (allowing the derivative of CPP to be calculated), peripheral arterial oxygen saturation (SaO_2), TCD measurement of the FV and SjO_2. In addition, I have introduced the novel methods of LDF and NIRS. It is the last two techniques on which my personal contribution has been concentrated, and so I will provide a brief introduction to these methods. For data concerning the analysis of TCD readings in head-injured patients, the reader is referred to our published data [14–17].

Laser Doppler Flowmetry

LDF is a technique which provides a continuous measure of relative microcirculatory flow [3, 18, 20, 27, 28, 33, 34]. The final signal generated is a measure of microcirculatory red cell flux (the product of red cell concentration and the red cell velocity). The theoretical basis for LDF is complex [2, 8, 60, 61, 81, 82]. Briefly, monochromatic coherent laser light, delivered via a transmitting fibre optic, is scattered by biological tissues. Light scattered from moving structures (red blood cells) experiences a Doppler shift in frequency (shifted light), whereas that reflected from surrounding stationary structures remains unaltered (reference light). The shifted and reference light signals are collected by a receiving afferent fibre optic and detected on the surface of a photodetector. The interference of the two signals produces optical beating (heterodyning), the frequency of which is equal to the Doppler-shifted frequency. A spectrum of shifted frequencies is generated from variations in red cell velocities and variations in the angle of incidence of light on red cell surfaces. The power spectral density of these shifted frequencies is determined by the red cell concentration and velocity. From the alternating photodetector current, various algorithms relating red cell flux to output signal can be derived [60, 61].

Experimental use of LDF in vitro and in vivo has consistently demonstrated a close linear correlation between LDF flux and CBF measured with a variety of standard methods, and the laser light used does not appear to alter the morphological and physiological characteristics of the vascular bed examined [24, 25, 62, 74, 77]. The method has shown particular use in the observation of changes in microcirculatory flow induced by physiological and pharmacological stimuli [78]. However, LDF is not quantitative, records from a small tissue volume and provides no information on the direction of blood flow. Further, experience has shown that the flux signal is very sensitive to the artefacts of local tissue pressure and movement, so that the reliability of the technique is critically dependent on the method of application [70]. Despite these drawbacks, LDF has already shown potential for blood flow measurements in several clinical disciplines, including neurosurgery [17, 46, 56, 57]. The advantage of LDF is that the technique provides a real-time measure of relative changes in capillary perfusion and can be put to advantage in the assessment of the microcirculatory response to a short-term therapeutic challenge.

Near Infrared Spectroscopy

NIRS is a non-invasive method which attempts to measure cerebral levels of oxyhaemoglobin (HbO_2) and deoxyhaemoglobin (Hb) by observing the absorption of near infrared light. The method has been used most extensively in the neonate, where inter-pterional transmission of light (transmission spectroscopy) can occur [11, 85, 87]. An absolute measure of changing brain haemoglobin saturation and blood volume is possible and has provided a means of monitoring the cerebrovascular response to certain therapeutic manipulations in critically ill infants [21].

In adults, scattering of light during passage through a greater thickness of tissue prevents adequate transmission of light to the opposite side of the skull [19, 22, 23]. Thus scattered light has to be sampled by a receiving probe placed ipsilateral to the source probe (reflectance spectroscopy). This results in limited topographical resolution, as it is not clear to what depth near infrared light penetrates the adult brain. Further, the thicker extracranial tissue will influence the sampled signal to a greater proportion when NIRS is used in adults, the significance of which remains unresolved [22]. Hence, although an estimate of the light path length transgressed is possible, the use of NIRS in the adult brain is presently considered non-quantitative. Despite these concerns, NIRS has been used to demonstrate predictable physiological changes in cerebral HbO_2 and Hb content during respiration [23], in response to various manoeuvres such as a carbon dioxide stress test [79] and in response to internal carotid artery cross-clamping during carotid endarterectomy [47].

Theory

Light at the near infrared end of the spectrum can penetrate the skull and is scattered within a composite of extra- and intracranial tissue [41]. The transmission of near infrared light through a scattering medium is given by the modified Beer-Lambert law:

$$OD = acLB + G$$

where OD is optical attenuation, a absorption coefficient (mM^{-1} cm^{-1}), c concentration of chromophore (mM), L light path length (cm), B factor relating tissue scattering and G factor relating tissue geometry.

Assuming that G remains constant, then relative changes in chromophore concentration can be expressed as:

$$\delta c = \delta OD / aLB$$

The coefficient a can be measured from lysed red cells in vitro, and B can be estimated in adults. Although L is unknown, it can be assumed to remain constant between measurements. Thus any change in OD is directly proportional to the change in chromophore concentration. Assuming that cerebral blood volume remains constant during recording, changes in HbO_2 and Hb will be equal and opposite, and an estimate of changing total Hb (tHb) can be calculated by simple summation of the respective signal changes.

Programme Objectives

The Neurosurgical Unit at Addenbrookes Hospital admits approximately 50 severely head-injured patients per year. We set out to employ the aforementioned techniques in a subset of patients who had received diffuse head injuries, who were without significant extracranial injuries and who did not require intracranial surgery. The purpose of this sub-selection was to identify those who were most likely to remain in the intensive care facility without excessive disturbance (such as transfer to theatre and radiological facilities) and in whom probe positioning would not pose a threat to the individual (such as those with excessive scalp trauma and swelling).

In this subgroup of head-injured patients, the objectives were as follows:
- To demonstrate the feasibility of applying multimodality monitoring throughout the period of ventilation
- To determine the reliability of the various parameters monitored
- To determine whether long-term monitoring can provide information regarding the relative pathophysiological state of the brain on a day-to-day basis
- To determine whether real-time monitoring can be employed to demonstrate the short-term pathophysiological response to a therapeutic manoeuvre (mannitol infusion for raised ICP)

Patients and Methods

These studies were approved by the Cambridge Local Research Ethics Committee.

Patients

Over a 24-month period, of 104 severely head-injured patients admitted to Addenbrookes Hospital, 36 patients (mean age, 26.6 years; range, 16–63 years; 12 males and 24 females) suffering diffuse closed head trauma with a Glasgow Coma Scale (GCS) score of 3–12 were considered suitable for multimodality monitoring of the cranial injury. Patients were selected on account of the absence of intracranial mass lesions requiring elevation of bone flaps, absence of extracranial trauma and scalp lacerations, which preclude safe application of surface probes (see below), absence of cervical neck injuries, absence of infection and clotting disorders and no prior internal jugular vein cannulation. All selected patients had probes positioned within 18 h of the injury.

Patient Management

All patients were sedated with midazolam (2–10 mg/h infusion) and fentanyl (0.1–0.5 mg/h infusion), paralysed with atracurium (0.3–1.2 mg/kg per h infusion), intubated and ventilated to a PCO_2 of 3.2–4.0 kPa. Intravenous fluid [Haemaccel (Hoechst) and normal saline] was administered to achieve a central venous pressure of between 5 and 10 cmH_2O. Attempts were made to maintain a CPP of greater than 55 mmHg in those patients with raised ICP using a constant infusion of dopamine (5–15 µg/kg per min). If this treatment failed, boluses of mannitol (200 ml of 20%, over 20 min) were given and repeated as necessary. Fluid status was monitored using a pulmonary artery catheter when considered necessary on clinical grounds.

Application of Long-Term Multimodality Monitoring

Cerebral Perfusion Pressure

Invasive and continuous monitoring of arterial blood pressure (20G catheters, Arrow, UK; transducers and monitors, S&W, Denmark) and ICP (Camino, USA) was routinely undertaken in all patients. The ICP-supporting bolt was positioned in the right or left frontal region according to the side of maximum injury, as seen on the admission CT scan. CPP was calculated from the digitised signals of mean arterial blood pressure (MABP) and ICP (see below).

Jugular Vein Oximetry

A 40 cm 4-French gauge fibre-optic catheter (Opticath, Abbott Laboratories, Chicago, USA) was placed into the internal jugular vein according to the methods of Andrews et al. [4], except that catheterisation was ipsilateral to the ICP and LDF probes. Jugular vein saturation was monitored using Oximetrix 3 (Abbott). In vivo calibration was carried out at the time of insertion using co-oximetry (Instruments Laboratory, IL 482, USA) and repeated every 8 h and whenever erroneous signals were suspected. The position of the catheter was checked radiologically.

Peripheral Oxygen Saturation

Peripheral saturation was recorded continuously with a pulse oximeter (Multinex monitoring).

Middle Cerebral Artery Flow Velocity

Continuous monitoring of FV was undertaken using a 2 MHz pulsed TCD (Scimed, Bristol, UK) probe insonating at a depth of 5.3–6.6 cm. The probe was attached to the scalp with an elasticated head band. Attending nurses were instructed on how to maintain an adequate FV signal following any patient manipulation.

Laser Doppler Flowmetry

At the time of insertion of the Camino ICP device, a second Camino bolt was sited approximately 3 cm further lateral to the ICP bolt to support a single LDF probe. Care was taken during the siting of this bolt not to breach the dura with the twist drill. Once in position, the dura was punctured with a lumbar needle passed down the bolt shaft. If any bleeding occurred, haemostasis was secured by irrigation with normal saline. A precalibrated and sterilised LDF probe was passed through the support bolt until the pliable surface of the cortex was encountered. With the probe connected to the monitor, the probe position was withdrawn (2–3 mm) until a maximal pulsatile signal was achieved. On further withdrawal (1–2 mm), the signal began to fall. The depth of the probe was increased again until the maximum signal was regained, at which point the locking screw was tightened. Repositioning of the probe was possible once the patient was in the neurointensive care unit, allowing intermittent optimisation of the signal. In four cases, intra-operative placement of the LDF probe indicated that the cortex had been breached (thereby offering little resistance to the LDF probe as it penetrated into the brain parenchyma). As the probe tip entered the brain parenchyma, the intensity of the signal fell to approximately 30% of the more superficial flux readings. To achieve a reliable surface cortical flux signal, these probes had to be resited.

Near Infrared Spectroscopy

NIRS (NIR 1000, Hamamatsu Photonic Ltd., Japan) was employed to allow non-invasive monitoring of relative changes in the chromophore levels of HbO_2 and Hb from the frontal region ipsilateral to the ICP and LDF probes. An estimate of absolute change in tHb can be derived from the simple summation of the raw HbO_2 and Hb signals. The optodes were placed on the forehead and frontal scalp with an intra-optode distance of 6 cm. One probe was sited on the forehead 2 cm above the supra-orbital ridge and 2 cm from the midline away from the sagittal sinus, and the second optode was positioned high on the frontal scalp (shaved if necessary) towards the coronal suture. Purpose-made light-occluding plastic caps were placed over each optode and secured with crepe bandage. Finally, the head was bound in a light-proof drape secured with adhesive tape. Once in place, the NIR 1000 was initiated and allowed to run undisturbed for 24 h. Extraneous stray light causes the sensitive photomultiplier tube (PMT) to switch off automatically, hence preventing further data collection until rectified. The probe positions require daily inspection to detect signs of evolving pressure sores. Raw data transfer to the recording hardware is via a RS232 with a maximum sampling rate of 2 Hz. Although an algorithm providing quantification of the signal changes in adults has been adopted in this study [11], it is the trend of NIRS signals which is reported. The machine is normalised every 4 h to compensate for signal drift.

Documentation of Nursing Events

For assistance with data analysis, the nursing staff were asked to document any events which might cause signal change or artefact (such as turning the patient, endotracheal suction, physiotherapy) or any change in therapeutic management (such as altering a dopamine infusion). They were also requested to perform their tasks during specific periods, providing 2-h intervals for undisturbed collection of data.

Signal Capture and Processing

For a detailed description of technical details of signal processing, the reader is referred to Czosnyka et al. [14]. Briefly, signals of MABP, ICP, SjO_2, arterial oxygen saturation (SaO_2), FV and LDF were sampled (frequency, 40 Hz), digitised (DT 2814, Data Translation, USA), filtered to remove high-frequency artefact and averaged over consecutive 3-s epochs. MABP and ICP were calibrated in appropriate units (mmHg). The raw LDF signal was recorded in arbitrary units (AU). In addition, NIRS data was transferred via a RS232, and although HbO_2 and Hb changes were initially recorded in AU, they were subsequently converted to quantified units of µmol/l according to the algorithm of Cope and Delpy [11].

Waveforms were processed using our specific software [14]. Data was stored on an IBM 386 portable PC. A minute by minute graphical display of mean CPP, ICP, LDF, FV, SjO_2, HbO_2 and Hb was provided to assist in the clinical management of the individual patients. Collection of data continued until the patient was withdrawn from the ventilator, had reached a static cerebral haemodynamic state or had died.

Data Analysis and Identification of Cerebral Events

The data from all patients were examined retrospectively using specific off-line software [14]. Cerebral events characterised by near synchronous changes in the various signals (Fig. 1) were marked, and the patient nursing records scrutinised to determine the clinical activity at that time. Events were recorded when there was a relative change in cerebral oxygenation (recorded by SjO_2 and/or NIRS), ICP, CPP and CBF (FV and/or LDF changes).

Data Analysis for Long-Term Monitoring of Superficial Cortical Perfusion

Time-averaged raw LDF data from patients in whom a reliable and continuous LDF signal had been recorded over at least 2 days ($n = 16$) was imported into a statistical package (Statgraphics 6+, Manugistics, USA), and the relationships between LDF signal and mean CPP were evaluated using analysis of variance (ANOVA) within a CPP range of 30–80 mmHg. Breakpoints for decreases in the LDF signals were defined at CPP levels below which the LDF signals started to decrease significantly ($p<0.05$).

Mannitol Infusion Studies

In fourteen diffusely head-injured patients, a total of 23 mannitol infusions were given when clinically indicated according to the patient management

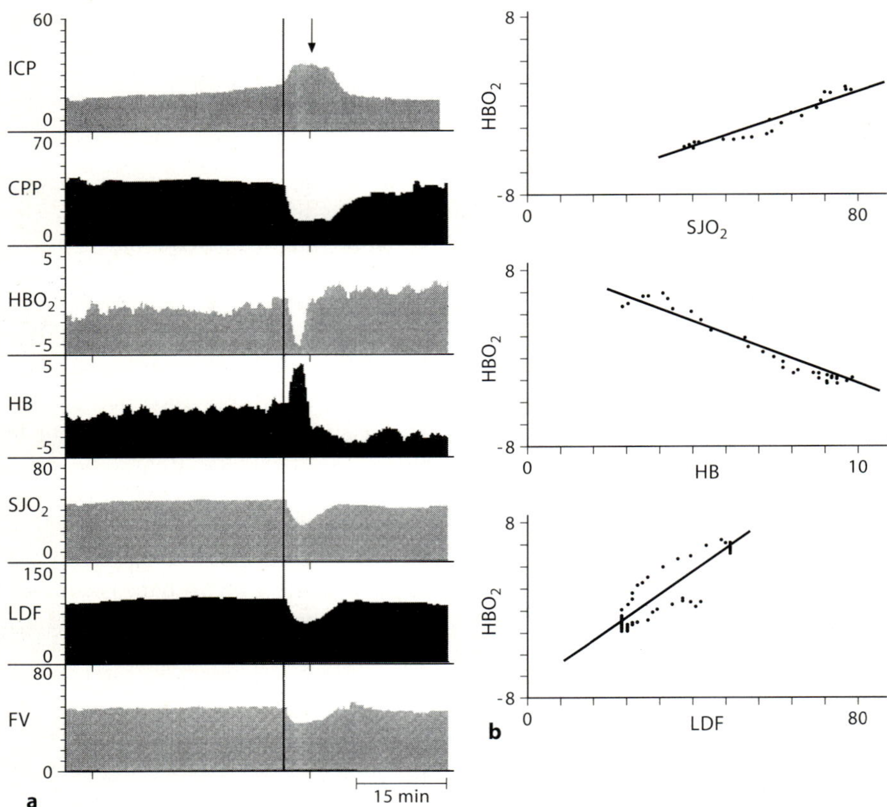

Fig. 1a,b. A spontaneous event recorded from the right side of the head in a 22-year-old with a diffuse head injury. Near infrared spectroscopy (NIRS) signals register a fall in HbO_2 (*arrow*) and a reciprocal rise in Hb, indicating haemoglobin desaturation. In this event, cerebral desaturation is confirmed by the fall in jugular vein oxygen saturation (*SjO_2*). *ICP*, intracranial pressure; *CPP*, cerebral perfusion pressure; *LDF*, laser Doppler flowmetry; *FV*, middle cerebral artery flow velocity

protocol. Variables collected were ICP, ABP, CPP, FV and LDF. Monitoring of brain oxygenation (NIRS and SJO_2) was not included at this stage of the programme.

After 30 min of baseline recordings, a single 200-ml bolus of normal saline was administered intravenously. After a further period of 30 min, a single 200-ml bolus of 20% mannitol was administered. In all cases, a 20-min infusion time was attempted. Throughout the recording, the patient was left undisturbed to reduce signal artefact and prevent probe displacement. Recordings were maintained for at least 30 min after completion of the mannitol bolus and continued provided there was no immediate need for medical or nursing manoeuvres. If any disturbance occurred, the recording was terminated.

Data Analysis

Time-averaged values for ABP, ICP, FV and LDF were calculated over 1-min periods at the following times during the infusion schedule: 10 min before start of infusion (baseline), at completion of infusion, 15 min after completion of infusion and 60 min after completion of infusion (mannitol only).

Values for CPP and FV Gosling pulsatility index (PI) were derived for the same epochs. In addition, the following indices of estimated cerebrovascular resistance (eCVR) were calculated:

$$eCVR\ (FV) = CPP/FV$$

and

$$eCVR\ (LDF) = CPP/LDF$$

In observing changes in raw LDF signal and subsequent calculation of eCVR (LDF), the biological zero (LDF signal value if CBF was stopped) is assumed to be zero. However, this probably introduces significant errors which result in underestimation of the proportional change in LDF and eCVR [70].

Assessment for Cerebral Autoregulation

Recordings prior to each mannitol infusion were reviewed, and the relationship between FV and CPP examined during natural variations in CPP. Those in which there was a close correlation ($r > 0.5$) were considered to demonstrate significantly disturbed autoregulation (non-autoregulating, NAR). Those with a correlation r less than 0.5 were considered to have intact autoregulation (AR) [15].

Statistical Analysis

The mean and standard error of the mean of the pooled data for each epochs after saline and mannitol infusions were calculated and plotted. Probability values were calculated using the paired t test. Analysis for the first single saline/mannitol run from each patient was initially gathered and probability values calculated (Table 1). A separate analysis for multiple runs in all patients (23 runs in 14 patients), AR (11 runs in nine patients) and NAR (12 runs in five patients) was also conducted.

Estimation of Duration of Effect for Mannitol

Normalised values for FV and LDF were plotted against time from the start of the infusion. A maximum response was identified after which the effect of mannitol decayed. An exponential model for the decay of effect was applied to allow calculation of the time constant.

Table 1. Maximum relative change (percentage increase over baseline) in variables following mannitol infusion

ABP (mmHg)	+1.7±6.5*
ICP (mmHg)	–21.0±18**
CPP (mmHg)	+10±15***
FV (cm/s)	+13±14****
PI	–2.9±7.7*****
LDF (arbitrary units)	+14±13******
eCVR-FV	–1.4±6.2*******
eCVR-LDF	–2.2±7.7*****

Values shown represent the average of the first mannitol run derived from each of the 14 patients.

ABP, arterial blood pressure; *ICP*, intracranial pressure; *CPP*, cerebral perfusion pressure; *FV*, flow velocity; *PI*, pulsatility index; *LDF*, laser Doppler flux; *eCVR*, estimated cerebrovascular resistance.

* $p=0.36$; ** $p=0.001$; *** $p=0.03$; **** $p<0.001$; ***** $p=0.39$; ****** p=0.002; ******* p=0.74.

Results

Long-Term Monitoring of Multiple Parameters and Capture of Cerebral Events

Signal Reliability

Complete multimodality monitoring was successfully achieved in 24 patients. A total of 1755 h of data was recorded (range, 4–185 h), of which 930 h (52%) was considered suitable for final analysis (mean, 26 h; range, 6–93 h). The commonest cause for data exclusion was suspected erroneous SjO_2 readings (47%) and automatic arrest of the NIRS signal due to stray light (33%). Other causes included arrest or significant damping of the ABP signal and misplacement of the TCD and LDF probes. The only signal that proved 100% reliable was that derived from the ICP probe.

Complications of Monitoring

There were no instances of intracranial haematoma or infection associated with the invasive ICP and LDF probes. In one patient, the bandages holding the NIRS probes were placed too tightly, causing a pressure sore which generated a permanent scar. Each probe is now examined daily to prevent a recurrence.

Event Recording

An example of a recorded event is shown in Fig. 1. In this patient, a plateau wave in ICP causes a severe fall in CPP to 15 mmHg. A relative fall in CBF and cortical perfusion is indicated by the synchronous decrease in FV and LDF. The event is also marked by the reciprocal changes in HbO_2 and Hb, indicating cerebral desaturation as confirmed by a fall in SjO_2. The close correlation between HbO_2 levels and the other variables suggests that the near infrared signal changes are largely derived from the intracranial compartment and probably reflect changes in regional cerebral oxygen saturation (see Appendix). Overall, 58 cerebral events were identified retrospectively in 16 patients (the median number of events per patient was two; range, none to 15). Each event lasted for a mean duration of 23.8 min (16.5–28.6 min; 95% CI range, 6–74 min). Forty-three (75%) of these events were associated with a mean fall in CPP of 22.8 mmHg, from 66 (62.4–70.7 mmHg) to 40.5 mmHg (34.2–48.9 mmHg). In the remaining 15 events, the mean CPP increased from 71.2 (61.0–84.8 mmHg) to 86.6 mmHg (72–108 mmHg).

Changes in Near Infrared Spectroscopy and Jugular Vein Oxygen Saturation Signals

Fifty-four events (94%) were accompanied by clear changes in the NIRS signals, whereas SjO_2 registered only 29 events (50%). Three discrete waves of increased ICP which compromised CPP led to synchronous drops in HbO_2, LDF and FV, whereas the SjO_2 monitor registered only the first event despite the CPP decreasing to below 30 mmHg in each case and the events being of similar duration. There were no instances in which similar NIRS profiles occurred without change in other monitored parameters.

Characterisation of Cerebral Events

Effect of Peripheral Desaturation. In 13 (20%) events, a fall in peripheral saturation to below 90% was recorded from seven patients in whom there were associated changes in HbO_2, Hb, FV and LDF. SjO_2 desaturation was seen in six of these events. An example of a recording is shown in Fig. 2. Two successive peripheral desaturations are seen with SaO_2 falling to 90% and 79%, respectively, but only the second resulted in a significant reciprocal fall in HbO_2 and a rise of Hb concentration, indicating cerebral desaturation. The increased magnitude of the second insult is also reflected by the rise in FV. SjO_2 showed no significant change. During a further episode of peripheral desaturation, changes in NIRS, FV and LDF occurred after the onset of peripheral desaturation by a mean time of 2.0 min (range, 0.6–3.8 min). In this case, HbO_2 and Hb both increased following recovery of peripheral oxygenation to above the pre-event baseline, suggesting reactive hyperaemia.

Intracranial Hypertension. In 19 events, a rise in ICP and fall in CPP preceded any change in HbO_2 and Hb by a mean time of 3.5 min (range, 2.6–4.8 min). SjO_2 changes were detected in ten of these events, which were synchronous with the NIRS. An example is shown in Fig. 3, in which an initial rise in ICP precedes the fall in HbO_2 and SjO_2. No change in tHb occurs during the active phase of the pressure wave.

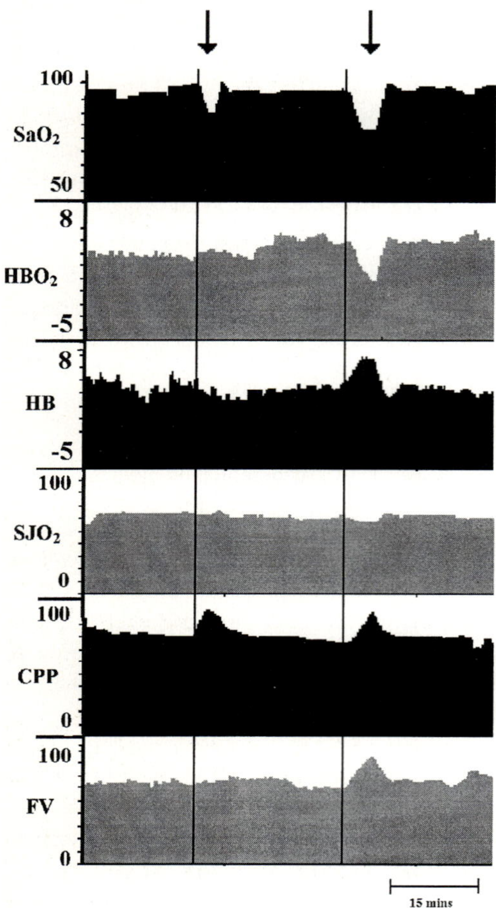

Fig. 2. One-hour recording from a 41-year-old head-injured man who developed pulmonary complications. Two successive episodes of peripheral desaturation are shown. In the second, the arterial oxygen saturation (SaO_2) falls to 79% and is accompanied by reciprocal changes in HbO_2 and Hb, whereas the jugular vein oxygen saturation (SjO_2) monitor failed to register this event. SaO_2, arterial oxygen saturation; *CPP*, cerebral perfusion pressure; *FV*, middle cerebral artery flow velocity

Intracranial Hyperaemia. Eleven events (six occurring in one patient) were recorded in five patients in which a synchronous rise in ICP, HbO_2, tHb, FV and LDF occurred. SjO_2 also increased in three of these events. The close correlation between the signal changes of all parameters suggests that the increased ICP was a consequence of rising CBF and cerebral blood volume.

Miscellaneous. Of the remaining 15 (26%) events, 11 were associated with a rise in ICP and fall in CPP, and one with a rise in CPP. Changes in HbO_2, HB, FV and LDF occurred without any significant time lag and were accompanied by SjO_2 changes in nine cases. The recordings in this group were complex, precluding

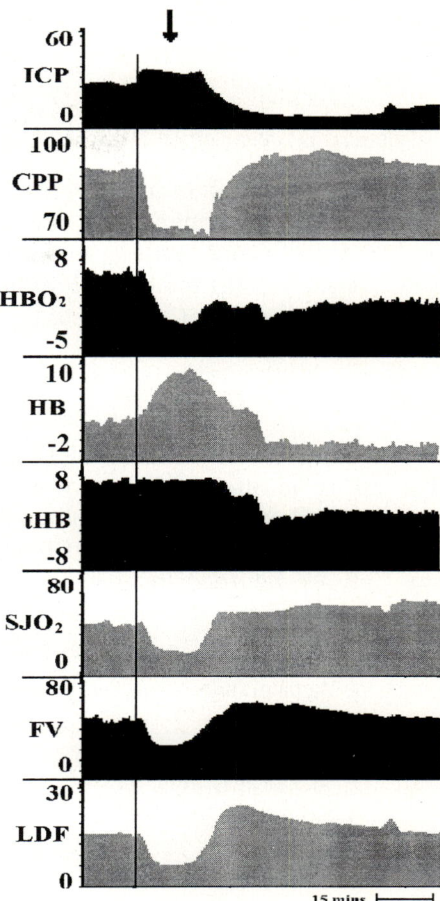

Fig. 3. Recording of an event characterised by intracranial hypertension with an increase in intracranial pressure (*ICP*) which lasted 14 min. This event was precipitated by turning the patient. Jugular vein oxygen saturation (*SjO$_2$*) monitoring confirms cerebral desaturation, as predicted from the reciprocal change in HbO$_2$ and Hb. After the wave of raised ICP passes, total Hb (*tHb*) reduces below baseline with improvement in the ICP, cerebral perfusion pressure (*CPP*) and SjO$_2$. *FV*, middle cerebral artery flow velocity; *LDF*, laser Doppler flowmetry

identification of the most likely cause. However, a high number ($n = 8$) of these events were associated with clinical procedures (see below).

Influence of Clinical Procedures

Although the majority of recorded events appeared spontaneously, 18 were associated with clinical and nursing procedures. Turning the patient led to a fall in CPP in eight cases, and changing the dopamine infusion syringe had a similar effect in four events with concomitant changes in NIRS and CBF signals. Finally, changing the ventilator setting caused a fall in peripheral saturation with cerebral desaturation in four events, and endotracheal suctioning caused complex increases in ICP in two cases.

Relationship Between Cortical Microcirculatory Flux and Cerebral Perfusion Pressure

Analysis of the relationship between raw LDF signal and CPP for 16 patients in whom long-term monitoring was achieved is shown in Fig. 4. The means and 95% confidence limits of the means for LDF signals at varying levels of CPP (30–80 mmHg) indicate a breakpoint of CPP (58 mmHg), at which LDF decreases with falling CPP ($p<0.05$).

Uncoupling Between Middle Cerebral Artery Flow Velocity and Laser Doppler Flowmetry Signals

Uncoupling between FV and LDF signal was seen in several instances, including during an attempted ween from dopamine, which caused a sudden increase in ICP and fall in CPP. Both FV and LDF signals fell simultaneously, indicating impaired perfusion. On restarting the dopamine and recovering the CPP, FV returned to previous levels, whereas LDF indicated a marked cortical hyperaemia lasting 25 min.

Effects of Mannitol Infusion on Cerebrovascular Perfusion

The mean duration of recording achieved before nursing or medical interruption was 56.3 min (range, 30–180 min) following the start of the mannitol in-

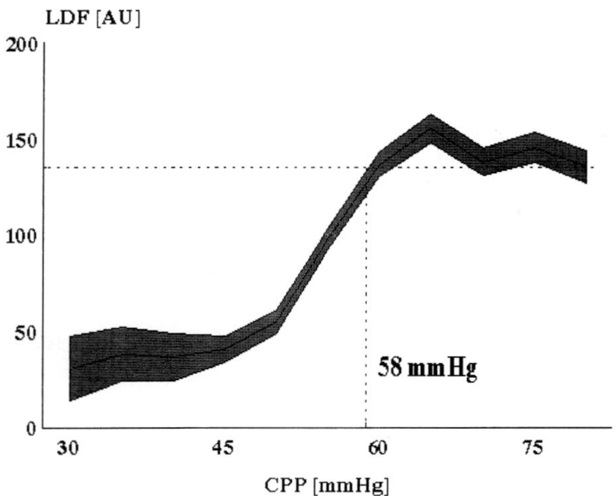

Fig. 4. Upper and lower limits of SE for the mean laser Doppler flowmetry (*LDF*) signal versus cerebral perfusion pressure (*CPP*) derived from the analysis of raw data from long-term recordings in 16 patients. The mean LDF signal shows a breakpoint at a CPP of 58 mmHg, below which cortical perfusion falls significantly ($p<0.05$)

fusion. The mean time taken to complete the infusions was 18.5 min for saline (range, 16.1–22.4 min) and 22.4 min for mannitol (range, 18.3–27.3 min). The maximum relative changes in variables following mannitol infusion are shown in Table 1.

Cerebral Perfusion Pressure

An increase in CPP was observed during and after the mannitol infusion in all patients (+10%, $p = 0.03$). This was seen in both AR (+9.1%) and NAR (+13.6%) subgroups. This resulted from a significant fall in ICP (–21%, $p = 0.001$; AR, –13%; NAR, –26.8%), whereas ABP was not significantly affected.

Middle Cerebral Artery Flow Velocity

A significant increase in FV was observed after mannitol infusion (+13.0%, $p < 0.001$) in both AR (+11.7%) and NAR (+19.4%) groups. The effect of mannitol on FV was maximal by the end of the bolus infusion and thereafter decayed in an exponential fashion, with an average time constant of 34.0 min. One AR patient showed an initial increase in FV after mannitol which fell to 21% below baseline at 50 min post-infusion.

There was a small decrease in eCVR-FV with mannitol (–1.4%, $p = 0.74$; AR, –5.5%; NAR, –0.2%).

Middle Cerebral Artery Flow Pulsatility Index

All patients showed a tendency to a fall in PI with mannitol (–2.9%, $p = 0.25$; AR, –0.4%; NAR, –10.5%).

Effects on Microcirculatory Perfusion

All patients showed a relative increase in LDF (+14.0%, $p = 0.002$) independent of autoregulatory status (AR, +12.5%; NAR, +21.5%). The maximum LDF response following mannitol was delayed (mean time from start of infusion, 30.5 min) compared to the effect on FV. Following the maximum response, the effect of mannitol on LDF decayed exponentially with a time constant of 38.0 min. No examples of post-infusion hypoperfusion were identified.

The calculated effect of mannitol on eCVR-LDF was a small decrease (–2.2%, $p = 0.39$; AR, –6.2%; NAR, –0.9%).

Saline

Saline produced a small fall in ICP (–8.0%; $p = 0.09$) which was associated with an small increase in CVR (CVR-FV, +6.2%, $p = 0.13$; CVR-LDF, +11.1%, $p = 0.12$). There was no other change in any parameter measured in any patient group.

Discussion

A technique for detecting cerebral ischaemic events in real time would be of considerable clinical value. Provisional experience indicates that this may be achieved in real time by the application of a computerised multimodality monitoring system. NIRS has demonstrated considerable promise as a non-invasive component, achieving high sensitivity compared to that of conventional invasive SjO_2 monitoring. Although still in a primitive format, authentic signal capture from all monitored parameters could be shown in 24 patients for 52% of the time. The intrusiveness of the equipment and computing was initially received badly among the intensive care staff. With time, nursing staff responded, and their contributions have helped to increase the proportion of time in which successful signal capture was obtained.

In view of my specific contributions to the components of NIRS and LDF, the first two sections of the discussion will focus on these two parameters and their potential use in clinical monitoring of head injured patients. The third section will discuss the use of multimodality monitoring for the analysis of a therapeutic challenge.

Near Infrared Spectroscopy

In reporting the early findings using NIRS in head-injured patients, I acknowledge the absence of quantified data. Rather, NIRS has been adopted purely as a trend monitor detecting relative changes in chromophore concentration by visual inspection of the recorded trend data files. The clinical relevance of these findings awaits improved reliability and a far wider experience with the technique. However, the high temporal resolution provided has already been used in a wide variety of ways [22, 23, 26, 31, 35, 38, 44].

Reliability

The employment of NIRS in the neurointensive care unit has posed problems. The prototype Hamamatsu 1000 is bulky, sensitive to variations in room temperature and exquisitely sensitive to outside light. As a result, probe application demands special attention, and it is necessary to bandage the scalp with light-proof drapes, which proved unpopular with the nursing staff and relatives. Despite these efforts, approximately one third of the data did not generate any NIRS recordings because of probe disruption and stray light interference. This difficulty has reduced with modified methods of probe application and occurs less frequently with the later version of the hardware (Hamamatsu NIR 500).

Signal Interpretation

The raw signals generated by NIRS sampling at 2 Hz can be noisy. The signals also display drift and are sensitive to movement artefact. Thus signal averaging is an essential part of the data processing. Because of drift, NIRS was adopted as a trend monitor only. However, drift over a 30- to 60-min period is very small when probe positioning is adequate, and so quantitative analysis of events over short (up to 1 h) durations are feasible and currently under evaluation. Once stabilised at a constant working temperature, most events are accompanied by obvious and dramatic changes in chromophore signals. The specificity for detecting events was high (94%) compared to SjO_2 monitoring (50%). The specificity also appeared high, as there was no instance in which NIRS registered obvious changes without accompanying ICP, CPP and relative CBF changes. Movement of the patient causing probe displacement caused obvious sudden changes in NIRS signals with no recovery. Although displaying high temporal resolution, event changes in NIRS evolved more gradually over several minutes, with recovery towards baseline after 20–60 min. The close correlation between NIRS signals and those derived from known intracranial parameters (FV, LDF and SjO_2) strengthens the opinion that the observed chromophore concentration changes are derived primarily from cerebral tissues.

Comparison of Near Infrared Spectoscopy with Jugular Vein Oxygen Saturation

NIRS demonstrated plausible changes in HbO_2 and Hb levels in approximately twice as many events as registered with SjO_2. The sensitivity and specificity of NIRS therefore appears high, but of course the clinical significance of these events remains unknown. Mixing of venous blood in the draining sinuses reduces the sensitivity of SjO_2 monitoring, which is generally regarded as a method of determining global cerebral desaturation. In contrast, the positioning of NIRS probes around the frontal region adjacent to the ICP and LDF probes allows monitoring of chromophore concentration changes from a small region of cortex. I therefore consider that, in many events, changes in HbO_2 and Hb reflect variations in global cerebral oxygenation.

Characterisation of Events

These observations confirm the diversity of events occurring within the traumatised brain. However, the high temporal resolution provided by the methods allows consideration of the most likely primary pathophysiological mechanisms responsible for a given event. Some patterns were encountered relatively frequently. Events following arterial desaturation were identified, since predictable changes in NIRS, CPP and haemodynamic parameters followed the fall in peripheral oxygen saturation by a mean time of 2 min. Not every episode of arterial desaturation caused intracranial events, and it is possible that cerebral changes occur only when desaturation falls below a threshold level and is sustained for a certain period of time. Verification of putative thresholds awaits further experience. Several events were seen in which the wave of raised ICP preceded any alteration in any other measured parameter by a mean time of 3.6 min. Subsequent changes in HbO_2, Hb,

SjO_2 and CBF were considered secondary to the fall in CPP. These events are typically accompanied by a fall in all signals, indicating a fall in blood volume (proportional to tHb) and CBF with consequent cerebral desaturation. The considerable time delay seen suggests the presence of oxygen and haemodynamic reserves which become depleted with prolonged reduction in CPP. Similar changes were recorded during events caused by temporary arrest of inotrope infusions during refilling of pump syringes.

In a small number of patients, hyperaemic episodes occur with increases in all measured parameters. The NIRS recordings seem to confirm the occurrence of episodes associated with increased blood flow and blood volume, and the close correlation between HbO_2, Hb, FV, LDF and ICP support the concept of associated vasodilation. Finally, in approximately one third of events, various responses were seen, with no clear time difference between parameters and no consistent pattern of change, which usually followed clinical manipulation of the patient. The complex recorded signal profiles may reflect superimposed factors, such as those accompanying endotracheal suctioning (causing raised ABP and ICP) to correct peripheral desaturation. The high number of events associated with clinical procedures is notable. Turning the patient was the commonest cause in this group and was probably related to inadequate positioning of the head. The sensitivity of CPP and cerebral oxygenation to inotropes is of potential concern, since once a patient is established on inotropic support, the fall in CPP resulting from planned or inadvertent withdrawal can be associated with dramatic changes in all measured parameters.

Summary

Unanswered questions surrounding the technique of NIRS in adult brain remain legion. Important issues such as quantification and spatial resolution were not addressed in this study. Rather, NIRS has been employed as a trend monitor in the Neurosurgical Intensive Care Unit to determine whether events could be detected by relative changes in levels of the chromophores HbO_2 and Hb. As such, clear signal changes associated with variations in ICP, CPP and CBF were found to occur, some of which may represent cerebral insults. Difficulties in long-term use of NIRS were experienced, but once the problems of probe application are overcome, NIRS shows promise as a monitor that warns of cerebral anoxic events with high sensitivity.

Laser Doppler Flowmetry

The advantage of LDF over other methods adopted for measurement of blood flow is the high temporal resolution provided [3, 6, 7, 17, 20, 25, 39, 46, 67, 68]. In cerebrovascular pathology, this facility is particularly important, since a fall in CBF lasting only a few minutes can cause irreversible ischaemic lesions. The potential use of LDF in monitoring cortical blood flow has been demonstrated in individual long-term recordings from 16 head-injured patients. Thus, by comparing variations in CPP with the flux signal, a real-time assessment of the autoregulatory state of the cortical microcirculation was possible. Further, such recordings may prove of value when considering general therapeutic manoeuvres to improve cortical flow (see below).

In most instances, changes in cortical perfusion measured with LDF were tightly coupled to changing FV. These findings lend support to the use of TCD in head-injured patients, indicating that variations in FV usually reflect variations of blood flow through the cortical microcirculation. However, uncoupling of FV and LDF signals were also noted. The hyperaemic response that followed manipulation of a dopamine infusion was registered only by LDF, indicating a possible differential effect of the drug on different parts of the vascular tree. A wider experience using combined TCD and LDF may help to determine the incidence and significance of such events where uncoupling occurs between large-vessel and small-vessel perfusion.

The technique of LDF is subject to several artefacts that are difficult to overcome in the clinical setting. Maintenance of constant probe position is particularly difficult. The sampling volume is small (1–2 mm^3) [2, 82] and may not give clinically relevant information in cases of focal pathology. Finally, LDF does not provide quantitative data. These points are considered further.

Artefact

By rigid fixation of a LDF probe in a position that samples from the surface of the brain, I have been able to record cortical red cell flux over long periods of time in ventilated head-injured patients. Such monitoring is only possible in paralysed patients, since movement significantly affects laser scatter, and hence output signal. Any movement incurred by nursing manoeuvres causes substantial variations in flux signal. The documentation of such events, and their restriction to allocated periods when possible, was an essential part of the study. Unfortunately, unlike recordings in experimental animals [70], LDF through the intact dura did not provide an adequate LDF signal in our patients (but recent increases with the laser power have overcome this difficulty). The probe was therefore positioned adjacent to the pia within the subdural space. The major concern regarding data collected using this arrangement is the effect of pressure on the cortex from an inflexible probe. Variations in cerebral swelling might impinge on the probe end, thereby reducing capillary perfusion in that area, and give an artificially low reading. However, no significant change in the LDF amplitude was noted in any recording during raised ICP. Further, adjusting the depth of probe penetration into the cranial cavity by 2–3 mm did not significantly affect the signal intensity. Additional penetration (5–6 mm) caused a fall in LDF output. I interpret this as indicating that the initial probe position in these patients was 2–4 mm above the cortical surface without significant impingement and that this position was maintained throughout the period of the recording.

At very low levels of CPP (<20 mmHg), LDF signals often became non-pulsatile and showed wide variations in signal intensity. These observations are likely to represent signal artefact resulting from mechanically induced oscillations in red cell movement and reverberant flow patterns. Since LDF cannot discriminate flow direction, excessively large signal changes result by summation.

Reliability

In six patients, the LDF signal proved unreliable despite frequent attempts to adjust the depth of probe penetration. A number of explanations can account for this. Firstly, the probe may have been overlying injured brain. Secondly, inadvertent breach of the cortical surface may cause local injury, which will impair red cell perfusion and cause local haemorrhage. Thirdly, the laser scatter theory of LDF assumes a small parenchymal concentration of red cells [60, 61]. Should the probe lie above a medium- or large-sized vessel, these assumptions are not satisfied. Finally, significant cerebral swelling may impair perfusion by the mechanisms outlined above. The fact that the probes were successfully re-sited in two patients indicates that attention to probe position with respect to the cortical surface is critical if LDF is to provide reliable data.

Sample Volume

A sample volume of 1–2 mm^3 indicates that LDF registers flow changes only within the cortical grey matter. Despite a restricted sample volume, the long-term recordings demonstrated the expected pathophysiological responses to raised ICP. Further, in cases where TCD recordings were also captured, a close correlation between FV and cortical perfusion was seen, indicating that changes in flow measured with LDF was representative of cortical perfusion in the general territory of the ipsilateral middle cerebral artery. Although LDF will not resolve focal anomalies in CBF, the technique may monitor general changes which are an important component of secondary mechanisms in brain injury. Inadvertent penetration of the pia during insertion often resulted in a drop of flux signal by up to 60%. This may reflect cortical injury, but may also indicate white matter flow. Sampling purely from the grey matter would seem an advantage, providing information on subpial collateral cortical flow. The flux values would also be devoid of multi-compartmental influences.

Quantification

Quantification of LDF has been hampered by the variation in baseline signals produced between readings. Our own observations using LDF in experimental animals has shown that, despite a very close correlation between cortical flux and CBF, the stable-state LDF baseline readings can vary considerably between animals. This partly results from variations in the "biological zero" output signal, which the instrument records when blood flow is zero [70]. In our head-injured patients, LDF signal levels for CPP above 65 mmHg were remarkably constant. Indeed, analysis of the raw LDF data has shown a clear autoregulatory break point at a CPP of 58 mmHg, below which cortical perfusion fails. This value is consistent with the autoregulatory breakpoint derived from FV waveform analysis obtained with TCD studies in other head-injured patients [15, 45]. This highly convergent data came as a surprise and indicates that the methodology adopted must provide a LDF baseline reading that is comparable between patients. One explanation is that the use of a skull bolt excludes external light, known to interfere with LDF, an arrangement not used in our experimental animals. Further, CBF values are known to be less variable in larger animals and less affected by influences of spreading depression. If further experience demonstrates reproducible flux signals in adult brain for a given CBF, reliable calibration of the LDF signal may prove possible.

Summary

In summary, early experience with LDF has indicated that long-term recordings of cortical perfusion are possible. The reliability of the technique appears to depend on probe positioning and avoidance of movement artefact. An autoregulatory threshold for cortical microcirculatory failure was demonstrated at a CPP of 58 mmHg, and variations in red cell flux were closely coupled with FV measurements in most, but not all instances. The high temporal resolution of LDF provides the opportunity to monitor the microcirculatory effects of therapy that alters the CPP in patients with raised ICP.

Use of Multimodality Monitoring for Observing the Response to Therapy – Mannitol Infusion Studies

The multimodality monitoring part of the programme examined the relative blood flow changes within different-sized cerebral vessels in response to an intravenous bolus of hypertonic mannitol and compared them to those occurring after isotonic normal saline. The findings show that significant haemorrheological changes follow mannitol administration, which can be effectively demonstrated in real time using multimodality bedside monitoring techniques. Mannitol, given over 20 min, causes a significant increase in relative CBF in both AR and NAR patients in which there is a tendency to a fall in the CVR.

Practical difficulties were encountered. In particular, ethical considerations prevented the protocol from continuing longer than 2 h without introducing potential interference from nursing and medical interventions. The recordings were stopped when the patient required repositioning or when further infusions were prescribed. Recent modifications to probe fixation have since allowed reliable recordings to occur long term, and so some of these early precautions may have been unnecessary. Nevertheless, the data obtained has allowed us to observe the early cerebral haemodynamic responses to saline and mannitol.

The consistent finding was an increase in FV and LDF, indicating a relative increase in CBF. Although the number of patients was small, this effect was apparent in both AR and NAR patients. The findings confirm that distinct haemodynamic changes occur after mannitol which may in part be responsible for the observed effects on ICP [52, 54, 80, 87]. It is of interest that these findings closely mirror those of Suzuki and Yoshisuji [83], who reported an increase in retinal blood flow after mannitol and (to a lesser extent) saline. Assuming a circulating blood volume of approximately 5–6 l, a 200 ml bolus will increase blood volume by only 3%–4%; the minimal effect of saline and mannitol on ABP when given slowly therefore comes as no surprise. Thus I consider that the changes in cerebral haemodynamic following mannitol were largely independent of ABP.

Relative Cerebral Blood Flow Changes

FV and microcirculatory red cell flux both increased after mannitol, a finding which has also been shown to occur in the experimental setting [36, 37, 40, 42, 55, 59, 75]. In the absence of changes in ABP, the relative increase in CBF could be explained by two possibilities: (1) mannitol induced cerebral vasodilation or (2) mannitol improved the flow characteristics of the blood, mainly by a rheological mechanism. The small decrease in PI, besides confirming a significant haemodynamic response, is not helpful in discriminating between these possibilities, since both would be expected to cause a fall in PI. However, vasodilation would increase ICP in patients with reduced intracranial compliance by virtue of an increased CBV. Early increases in CBV have been reported after rapid mannitol infusion, but these were associated with an increased ICP [65, 66]. Since this was not seen in our clinical subgroup, these findings support the opinion that the fall in CVR is primarily due to improved blood rheology. The effect of mannitol in reducing blood viscosity is well known and was not re-examined in this study [5, 37, 58, 69].

The finding that relative CBF increased in AR head-injured patients contrasts with the classical studies by Muizelaar et al. [58], who demonstrated increased CBF in the NAR subgroup only. Furthermore, the tendency to a fall in CVR in AR patients and the fall in PI is not in keeping with the proposals that mannitol causes significant vasoconstriction secondary to "viscosity autoregulation". In making this comparison, I acknowledge that the present data is derived from a far smaller pilot group of patients and that the prime purpose of the study was the assessment of the multimodality method for analysing a therapeutic agent. Further, formal identification of the pressure autoregulatory status (by induction of hypo- or hypertension) was not conducted in our patients. Instead, I relied upon observing the changing baseline relationship between relative CBF and CPP, which allows an estimation of autoregulatory status [15]. Including the data of several runs from the same patient may also direct the results inappropriately in the subgroup analysis. Netherthless, it was clear that all mannitol infusions in all patients caused relative increases in CBF.

The different times at which a maximal effect was detected on FV and LDF are difficult to explain. In contrast, the time constants describing the exponential decay of effect are almost identical. Methodological factors may be responsible. LDF precludes absolute quantification, since it is not possible to estimate the biological zero in the present clinical setting [70]. This may in part explain the proportional differences of mannitol effect on LDF signals compared to FV. Since LDF averages flux signal changes from an estimated volume of cortex of 1–2 mm^3, the technique (in the present format) may be unable to resolve heterogenous patterns in microcirculatory perfusion. Improved blood flow characteristics encouraging shunting through anatomically and physiologically favourable channels may not be detected with LDF. Finally, since haemorrheological changes may have differential effects on laminar flow through large vessels compared to non-laminar flow through a microvascular bed, the correlation between FV and LDF under changing conditions of rheology may not be linear. Indeed, the phenomenon of uncoupling between LDF and FV in head-injured patients has already been highlighted (see above) [46].

Effects on Intracranial Pressure

The effect of mannitol on ICP was large and associated with a tendency to decreased CVR. The data therefore supports the notion that mannitol increases CBF by reducing CVR, and this is most likely due to reduced blood viscosity. One cannot exclude a vasoconstrictive element as postulated by others [58], but in the face of a fall in CVR I feel that this is unlikely to be the primary cause of a fall in ICP. Rather, I prefer the concept that the reduced CVR encourages fluid transudation into the intravascular space by reducing the hydrostatic pressure operating across the microvascular wall. The free water content in the extracellular spaces is high compared to the intracellular compartments, hence movement of freely diffusible water across the microvascular membranes. In a state of reduced intracranial compliance, the effect of a relatively small reduction in extracellular volume in ICP may be considerable and rapid. This mechanism is therefore feasible.

Future Applications of Middle Cerebral Artery Flow Velocity and Laser Doppler Flowmetry Measurements

The use of non-invasive techniques to assess the cerebral haemodynamic changes occurring with therapy is not new. Thiel et al. [84] demonstrated the different effects of volatile anesthetic agents on FV by showing an increase in relative CBF with halothane, but not enflurane or isoflurane. The study of effects of mannitol on CBF intra-operatively using LDF has also been described in single patients [25]. However, the use of multiple modality methods has not yet received wide attention. While I acknowledge that some of the present findings are confirmatory, they were achieved without involving transfer to expensive facilities for imaging purposes. In addition, the methods generate real-time information allowing rapid interpretation. I therefore envisage a role for bedside multimodality monitoring in deciphering mechanisms of drug effect and for assisting in the identification of candidates who are the most likely to respond to specific therapies influencing cerebrovascular haemodynamics.

Summary

A mannitol bolus administered to diffusely head-injured patients causes a rise in relative CBF detected in the middle cerebral artery and in the microcirculation in real time, a rise which does not occur after isotonic saline. The use of the bedside multimodality method to monitor neurointensive patients allows rapid identification of changing cerebral haemodynamics and appears to offer a useful means of studying the effects of agents that change intracranial blood flow.

Concluding Remarks

Initial experience with bedside multimodality monitoring has been encouraging. It appears possible to apply multimodality monitoring throughout the period of ventilation with a global signal reliability of approximately 50%. This will no doubt improve as experience with application accumulates and as probe design improves. In addition, provided that great care is taken in positioning the sampling probe, the data concerning LDF over several days indicates that long-term monitoring providing information regarding the relative pathophysiological state (e.g. failure of cortical autoregulation) of the brain can be achieved on a day-to-day basis. This compliments our parallel work on real-time waveform analysis of TCD FV signals [15–17].

Attempts to assess these patients have led us to consider the problem with a greater pathophysiological understanding in each individual case, allowing a more informed response and targeted therapy. The monitors have also indirectly provoked an increase awareness on the unit such that supporting staff have become more vigilant in their reporting of possible adverse events. It is my own impression that the care of the head-injured patent in Addenbrookes Hospital has improved as a result, although this statement awaits the outcome of the East Anglian Regional Head Injury Audit. The referral of head-injured patients has also increased as a consequence of the increasing perception of the need for monitoring in comatose patients. The practicalities of providing this service clearly need addressing. I believe that, as experience accumulates, certain modalities will emerge, providing the key information of clinical importance. The system can then be trimmed for simplicity and increased reliability, at which point a wider clinical application can be considered.

Future Intentions

In collaboration with Hamamatsu Photonics and the Department of Biomedical Engineering at University College in London (Professor D. Delpy and colleagues), we have been given the opportunity to calibrate a spatially resolved spectroscope (SRS). Our provisional experience using NIRS in patients undergoing carotid endarterectomy led to the design of a provisional algorithm, which has been incorporated into the prototype version of the SRS [1]. We are now using the SRS to observe events of cerebral desaturation in head-injured patients and in those undergoing cardiac bypass surgery. It is our intention to capture high-quality data to allow the provision of the definitive algorithm for a commercial version of the SRS. We consider that this technology may be of considerable clinical importance and is therefore central to our present objectives.

The other main ongoing projects involve the multimodality assessment of novel neuroprotective agents. Both Bosentan (an endothelin-α and -β receptor blocker) and N-acetyl cysteine (an anti-oxidant used for treating patients with hepatic failure) are presently under evaluation in coma producing subarachnoid haemorrhage and head injury, respectively. Should these agents produce short-term improvements in the different haemodynamic indices measured (surrogate end points), then trials that test clinical efficacy can be considered.

Our long-term objectives are to introduce computer-guided treatments into the neurointensive care unit. Our experience in the laboratory have shown that sophisticated computer systems can be used to maintain different levels of blood pressure with a high degree of stability by directing mechanical infusion/exfusion pumps [2]. Such facilities can be potentially of use in comatous patients, e.g. to maintain a constant CPP. Thus, if raised ICP compromises CPP, signal analysis of the multiple variables can allow the most appropriate therapeutic response in an almost immediate fashion (mannitol and/or inotrope and/or vasoconstrictors), and continued signal surveillence may prevent inappropriate or excessive therapy and rebound phenomena.

Acknowledgments. I am indebted to my colleagues and collaborators for their help and encouragement during this period of development. Dr. Marek Czosnyka, Piotre Smielewski, and Professor John Pickard have been central to my work. I am also grateful to the nursing staff on the Neurointensive Care Unit, and to those supporting the neurosurgical theatres, for their patience and co-operation.

Appendix

The following mathematical considerations show that, providing Hb is changing in inverse proportion to HbO_2 (negative linear correlation), changes in haemoglobin saturation can be expected to vary in proportion to HbO_2. Regional haemoglobin saturation (HbSat) may be expressed in terms of Hb and HbO_2 concentrations:

$$HbSat = \frac{HbO_2}{HbO_2 + Hb} \tag{1}$$

Assuming that, in a given time period Hb and HbO_2 show negative linear correlation, the changes in Hb can be expressed as follows:

$$\Delta Hb = -k \times HbO_2 \tag{2}$$

where k is an positive proportionality factor. If changes in Hb and HbO_2 are relatively small, the following approximation can be applied:

$$\Delta HbSat \approx \frac{\delta HbSat\,(Hb,\ HbO_2)}{\delta HbO_2} \times \Delta HbO_2 + \frac{\delta HbSat\,(Hb,\ HbO_2)}{\delta Hb} \times Hb \tag{3}$$

Substituting Eq. 1 into Eq. 3, the following relation is obtained:

$$\Delta HbSat \approx \frac{(Hb \times \Delta HbO_2)}{(Hb + HbO_2)^2} - (HbO_2 \times \Delta Hb) \tag{4}$$

Now, substituting Eq. 2 into Eq. 4, the relation between HbSat and HbO_2 is obtained:

$$\Delta HbSat \approx \Delta HbO_2 \times \frac{(Hb + k \times HbO_2)}{(Hb \times HbO_2)^2} = \Delta HbO_2 \times const. \tag{5}$$

Thus changes in the haemoglobin saturation vary in proportion to changes in HbO_2, with the proportionality factor dependent on the baseline values of Hb and HbO_2 and the regression coefficient k. Note that if reciprocal Hb and HbO_2 changes occur such that the tHb content remains constant, the proportionality factor is equal to the reciprocal of tHb. Figure 1b shows an example of the relation between Hb, HbO_2 and SjO_2. Hb and HbO_2 show an proportional inverse relation. Therefore, from the above, HbSat should change in proportion to HbO_2. Further, assuming that the metabolic rate remains constant and changes in HbSat reflect variations in global brain oxygenation saturation, the SjO_2 values should follow variations in regional cerebral oxygen saturation – hence the linear positive correlation between HbO_2 and SjO_2.

References

1. Aaslid R, Lundar T, Lindegaard KF, Nornes H (1986) Estimation of cerebral perfusion pressure and transcranial Doppler recordings. In: Miller JD, Teasdale GM et al (eds) Intracranial pressure, vol VI. Springer, Berlin Heidelberg New York
2. Ahn H, Johansson K, Lundgren O, Nilsson GE (1987) In vivo calibration of signal processors for laser Doppler tissue flowmeters. Med Biol Eng Comput 25:207–211
3. Almond NE, Wheatley AM (1992) Measurement of hepatic perfusion in rats by laser Doppler flowmetry. Am J Physiol 262:G203-209
4. Andrews PJD, Dearden NM, Miller JD (1991) Jugular bulb cannulation: description of a cannulation technique and validation of a new continuous monitor. Br J Anaes 67:553–558
5. Andrews RJ, Bringas BS, Muto RP (1993) Effects of mannitol on cerebral blood flow, blood pressure, blood viscosity, hematocrit, sodium and potassium. Surg Neurol 39:218–222
6. Arbit E, DiResta GR, Bedford et al (1989) Intraoperative measurement of cerebral and tumour blood flow with laser Doppler flowmetry. Neurosurgery 24:166–170
7. Bonard D, Bounameaux H, Fagrell B (1992) Effects of oxygen inhalation on skin microcirculation in patients with peripheral arterial occlusive disease. Circulation 86:878–86
8. Bonner R, Nossal R (1981) Model for laser Doppler measurements of blood flow in tissue. Appl Optics 20:2097–2107
9. Bouma GJ, Muizelaar PJ, Stringer WA et al (1992) Ultra-early evaluation of regional cerebral blood flow in severely head injured patients using xenon-enhanced computerised tomography. J Neurosurg 77:360–368
10. Chan KH, Miller JD, Dearden NM et al (1992) The effect of changes in cerebral perfusion pressure upon middle cerebral artery blood flow velocity and jugular bulb venous oxygen saturation after severe brain injury. J Neurosurg 77:55–61
11. Cope M, Delpy DT (1988) A system for long term measurement of cerebral blood and tissue oxygenation in newborn infants by near infrared transillumination. Med Biol Eng Comp 26:289–294
12. Cruz J, Miner ME, Allen SJ et al (1991) Continuous monitoring of cerebral oxygenation in acute brain injury: assessment of cerebral hemodynamic reserve. Neurosurg 29:743–749
13. Cruz J (1993) On-line monitoring of global cerebral hypoxia in acute brain injury. Relationship to intracranial hypertension. J Neurosurg 79:228–233
14. Czosnyka M, Whitehouse H, Smielewski P et al (1994) Computer supported multimodal monitoring in neuro intensive care. Int J Clin Monitor Comput 11:223–232
15. Czosnyka M, Guazzo E, Iyer V et al (1994) Testing of cerebral autoregulation in head injury by waveform analysis of blood flow velocity and cerebral perfusion pressure. Acta Neurochir Suppl 60:468–471
16. Czosnyka M, Kirkpatrick P, Guazzo E et al (1994) Can TCD pulsatility indices be used for a non-invasive assessment of cerebral perfusion pressure in head injured patients? In: Nagai H, Kamiya K, Ishii S (eds) Intracranial pressure, vol IX. Springer, Berlin Heidelberg New York, pp 146–149
17. Czosnyka M, Richards H, Kirkpatrick P, Pickard J (1994) Assessment of cerebral autoregulation using ultrasound and laser doppler waveforms – an experimental study in anaesthetized rabbits. Neurosurgery 35:287–293
18. Davies EG, Sullivan PM, Fitzpatrick M, Kohner EM (1992) Validation and reproducibility of bidirectional laser Doppler velocimetry for the measurement of retinal blood flow. Current Eye Res 11:633–640
19. Delpy DT, Cope M, van der Zee P et al (1988) Estimation of optical pathlength through tissues by direct time of flight measurement. Phys Med Biol 33:1433–1442
20. Dirnagl U, Kaplan B, Jacewicz M, Pulsinelli W (1989) Continuous measurement of cerebral blood flow by laser Doppler flowmetry in a rat stroke model. J Cereb Blood Flow Metabol 9:589–596

21. Edwards AD, McCormick DC, Roth SC et al (1992) Cerebral hemodynamic effects of treatment with modified natural surfactant investigated by near infrared spectroscopy. Pediatr Res 32:532–536

22. Elwell CE, Cope M, Edwards AD et al (1992) Measurement of cerebral blood flow in adult humans using near infrared spectroscopy – methodology and possible errors. Adv Exp Med Biol 317:235–245

23. Elwell CE, Owen-Reece H, Cope M et al (1993) Measurement of changes in cerebral haemodynamics during inspiration and expiration using near infrared spectroscopy. Adv Exp Med Biol 245:619–626

24. Eyre JA, Essex JTH, Flecknell PA et al (1988) A comparison of measurements of cerebral blood flow in the rabbit using laser Doppler spectroscopy and radionuclide labelled microspheres. Clin Phys Physiol Meas 9:65–74

25. Fasano VA, Urciuoli R, Bolognese P, Mostert M (1988) Intraoperative use of laser Doppler in the study of cerebral microvascular circulation. Acta Neurochir 95:40–48

26. Ferrari M, Zannetta E, Giannini I et al (1986) Effects of carotid compression test on regional cerebral blood volume, haemoglobin oxygen saturation and cytochrome-c-oxidase redox level in cerebrovascular patients. Adv Exp Med Biol 200:213–222

27. Florence G, Seylaz J (1992) Rapid autoregulation of cerebral blood flow: a laser-Doppler flowmetry study. J Cereb Blood Flow Metab 12:674–680

28. Goadsby PJ (1991) Characteristics of facial nerve elicited cerebral vasodilation determined using laser Doppler flowmetry. Am J Physiol 260:R255-262

29. Goncalves JM, Vaz R, Cereo A et al (1994) HM-PAO SPECT in head trauma. Acta Neurochir [Suppl] 55:11–13

30. Gopinath PS, Robertson CS, Contant CF et al (1994) Jugular venous desaturation and outcome after head injury. J Neurol Neurosurg Psychiatry 57:717–723

31. Gopinath PS, Robertson CS, Grossman RG, Chance B (1993) Near infrared spectroscopic localof intracranial hematomas. J Neurosurg 79:43–47

32. Grosset DG, Strebel S, Straiton J et al (1993) Impaired carbon dioxide reactivity predicts poor outcome in severe head injury: a transcranial Doppler study. In: Avezaat CJJ, van Eijndhoven JHM, Maas AIR, Tans JTJ (eds) Intracranial pressure, vol VIII. Springer, Berlin Heidelberg New York, pp 322–326

33. Haberl RL, Heizer ML, Ellis EF (1989) Laser-Doppler assessment of brain microcirculation: effect of systemic alterations. Am J Physiol 256:H1247-H1254

34. Haberl RL, Heizer ML, Ellis EF (1989) Laser-Doppler assessment of brain microcirculation: effect of local alterations. Am J Physiol 256:H1255-H1260

35. Hampson NB, Camporesi EM, Stolp BW et al (1990) Cerebral oxygen availability by NIRS spectroscopy during transient hypoxia in humans. J Appl Physiol 69:907–913

36. Harada K, Hayashi T, Anegawa S (1993) Effect of rapid mannitol infusion on middle cerebral artery blood flow velocity and pulsatility index – a transcranial Doppler ultrasonography study in monkeys. Brain Nerve 45:649–654

37. Harrison MJ (1989) Influence of hematocrit in the cerebral circulation. Cerebrovasc Brain Metabol Rev 1:55–67

38. Hoshi Y, Tamura M (1993) Detection of dynamic changes in cerebral oxygenation coupled to neuronal function during mental work in man. Neurosci Lett 150:5–8

39. Iadecola C, Reis D (1990) Continuous monitoring of cerebrocortical blood flow during stimulation of the cerebellar fastigial nucleus: a study by laser Doppler flowmetry. J Cereb Blood Flow Metab 10:608–617

40. Jafar JJ, Johns LM, Mullan SF (1986) The effect of mannitol on cerebral blood flow. J Neurosurg 64:754–759

41. Jobsis FF (1977) Noninvasive, infrared monitoring of cerebral and myocardial oxygen suffciency and circulation parameters. Science 198:1264–1267

42. Johnston IH, Harper AM (1973) The effect of mannitol on cerebral blood flow. An experimental study. J Neurosurg 38:461–471

43. Jones PA, Andrews PJD, Midgley S et al (1993) Assessing the burden of secondary insults in head injured patients during intensive care. J Neurol Neurosurg Psychiatry 56:571–572

44. Kato T, Kamei A, Takashima S, Ozaki T (1993) Human visual cortical function during photic stimulation monitoring by means of near infrared spectroscopy. J Cereb Blood Flow Metab 13:516–520

45. Kirkpatrick PJ, Czosnyka M, Pickard J (1995) Multimodality monitoring in neurointensive care. J Neurol Neurosurg Psychiatry 60:131–139

46. Kirkpatrick PJ, M Czosnyka, P Smielewski et al (1994) Continuous monitoring of cortical perfusion using Laser Doppler flowmetry in ventilated head injured patients. J Neurol Neurosurg Psychiatry 57:1382–1388

47. Kirkpatrick PJ, Smielewski P, Whitfield P et al (1995) An observational study of near infrared spectroscopy during carotid endarterectomy. J Neurosurg 82:756–763

48. Kirkpatrick PJ, Smielewski P, Czosnyka M, Menon DA, Pickard JD (1995) Near infrared spectroscopy in head injured patients. J Neurosurg 83:963–970

49. Macpherson P, Graham DI (1973) Arterial spasm and slowing of the cerebral circulation in the ischaemia of head injury. J Neurol Neurosurg Psychiatry 48:560–564

50. Marion DW , Darby J, Yonas H (1991) Acute regional cerebral blood flow changes caused by severe head injuries. J Neurosurg 74:407–414

51. Marmarou A, Anderson RL, Ward JD et al (1991) Impact of ICP instability and hypotension in patients with severe head trauma. J Neurosurg 75:859–866

52. Marshall LF, Smith RW, Rauscher LA, Shapiro HM (1978) Mannitol dose requirements in brain-injured patients. J Neurosurg 48:169–172

53. Mass AIR, Fleckenstein W, De Jong DA, Wolf M (1993) Effect of increased ICP and decreased cerebral perfusion pressure ion brain tissue and cerebrospinal fluid oxygens tension. In: Avezaat CJJ, van Eijndhoven JHM, Maas AIR, Tans JTJ (eds) Intracranial pressure, vol VIII. Springer, Berlin Heidelberg New York, pp 233–237

54. Mendelow AD, Teasdale GM, Russell T, Flood J, Patterson J, Murray GD (1985) Effect of mannitol on cerebral blood flow and cerebral perfusion pressure in human head injury. J Neurosurg 63:43–48

55. Meyer FB, Anderson RE, Sundt TM, Yaksh TL (1987) Treatment of experimental focal cerebral ischemia with mannitol. Assessment by intracellular brain pH, cortical blood flow, and electroencephalography. J Neurosurg 66:109–115

56. Meyerson BA, Gunasekera L, Linderoth B, Gazeliu B (1991) Bedside monitoring of regional cortical blood flow in comatose patients using laser Doppler flowmetry. Neurosurgery 29:750–755

57. Muir JK, Boerschel M, Ellis EF (1992) Continuous monitoring of postraumatic cerebral blood flow using laser-Doppler flowmetry. J Neurotrauma 9:355–362

58. Muizelaar JP, Lutz III HA, Becker DP (1984) Effect of mannitol on ICP and CBF and correlation with pressure autoregulation in severely head-injured patients. J Neurosurg 61:700–706

59. Muizelaar JP, Wei EP, Kontos HA, Becker DP (1983) Mannitol causes compensatory cerebral vasoconstriction and vasodilation in response to blood viscosity changes. J Neurosurg 59:822–828

60. Nilsson GE, Tenland T, Oberg PA (1980) Evaluation of a laser Doppler flowmeter of tissue blood flow. Trans Biomed Engineer 27:579–604

61. Nilsson GE (1984) Signal processors for laser Doppler tissue flowmeters. Med Biol Eng Comput 22:343–348

62. Nobes MS, Harris PJ, Yamanda H, Mendelsohn FA (1991) Effects of angiotensin on renal cortical and papillary blood flows measured by laser-Doppler flowmetry. Am J Physiol 261:F998-1006

63. Obrist WD, Wilkinson WE (1990) Regional cerebral blood flow measurement in humans by xenon-133 clearance. Cerebrovasc Brain Metabol Rev 2:283–327

64. Pickard JD, Czosnyka M (1993) Management of raised intracranial pressure. J Neurol Neurosurg Psychiatry 56:845–858

65. Ravussin P, Archer DP, Tyler JL, Meyer E, Abou-Madi M, Diksic M, Yamamoto L, Trop D (1986) Effects of rapid mannitol infusion on cerebral blood volume. A positron emission tomographic study in dogs and man. J Neurosurg 64:104–113

66. Ravussin P, Abou-Madi M, Archer D, Chiolero R, Freeman J (1988) Changes in CSF pressure after mannitol in patients with and without elevated CSF pressure. J Neurosurg 69:869–876
67. Rendell M, Bergman T, O'Donnell G et al (1989) Microvascular blood flow, volume, and velocity measured by laser Doppler techniques in IDDM. Diabetes 38:819–824
68. Rosenblum BR, Bonner RF, Oldfield EH (1987) Intraoperative measurement of cortical blood flow adjacent to cerebral AVM using laser Doppler velocimetry. J Neurosurg 66:396–399
69. Rosner MJ, Coley I (1987) Cerebral perfusion pressure: a hemodynamic mechanism of mannitol and the postmannitol hemogram. Neurosurgery 21:147–156
70. Richards HK, Czosnyka M, Kirkpatrick P, Pickard JD (1995) Estimation of laser Doppler flux biological zero using basilar artery flow velocity in the rabbit. Am J Physiol 268:H213–H217
71. Robertson CS, Contant CF, Gokaslan ZL et al (1992) Cerebral blood flow, arteriovenous oxygen difference, and outcome in head injured patients. J Neurol Neurosurg Psychiatry 55:594–603
72. Robertson CS, Simpson RK Jr (1991) Neurophysiologic monitoring of patients with head injuries. Neurosurg Clin North Am 2:285–299
73. Sheinberg M, Kanter MJ, Robertson CS, et al (1992) Continuous monitoring of jugular venous oxygen saturation in head-injured patients. J Neurosurg 76:212–217
74. Shepherd AP, Riedel GL, Kiel JW et al (1987) Evaluation of an infrared laser Doppler blood flowmeter. Am J Physiol 252:G832–839
75. Shirane R, Weinstein PR (1992) Effect of mannitol on local cerebral blood flow after temporary complete cerebral ischemia in rats. J Neurosurg 76:486–492
76. Sjeso BK (1992) Pathophysiology and treatment of focal cerebral ischaemia, parts I and II. J Neurosurg 77: 169–184, 337–354
77. Skarphedinsson JO, Harding H, Thoren P (1988) Repeated measurements of cerebral blood flow in rats. Comparisons between the hydrogen clearance method and laser Doppler flowmetry. Acta Physiol Scand 134:133–142
78. Skarphedinsson JO, Delle M, Hoffman P, Thoren P (1989) The effects of naloxone on cerebral blood flow and cerebral function during relative cerebral ichaemia. J Cereb Blood Flow Metab 9:515–522
79. Smielewski P, Kirkpatrick PJ, Minhas P et al (1995) Can cerebrovascular reactivity be measured using near-infrared spectroscopy. Stroke 25:225–229
80. Smith HP, Kelly DL, McWhorter JM (1986) Comparison of mannitol regimens in patients with severe head injury undergoing intracranial monitoring. J Neurosurg 65:820–824
81. Stern MD (1975) In vivo evaluation of microcirculation by coherent light scattering. Nature 254:56–58
82. Stern MD, Lappe LD, Bowen PD (1977) Continuous measurement of tissue blood flow by laser-Doppler spectroscopy. Am J Physiol 232:H441–H448
83. Suzuki Y, Yoshiisji M (1994) Effect of mannitol on human retinal blood flow. Acta Soc Ophthal Japonica 98:1005–1009
84. Thiel A, Zickmann B, Zimmermann R, Hempelmann G (1992) Transcranial Doppler sonography: effects of halothane, enflurane and isoflurane on blood flow velocity in the middle cerebral artery. Br J Anaeth 68:388–393
85. van der Zee P, Cope M, Arridge SR et al (1992) Experimentally measured optical pathways for the adult head, calf and forearm of the newborn infant as a function of interoptode spacing. Adv Exp Med Biol 316:143–153
86. Wise BL, Chater N (1962) The value of hypertonic mannitol solution in decreasing brain mass and lowering cerebrospinal-fluid pressure. J Neurosurg 19:1038–1043
87. Wyatt JS, Cope M, Delpy DT et al (1986) Quantification of cerebral oxygenation and haemodynamics in sick newborn infants by near infrared spectrophotometry. Lancet ii:1063–1066

Miscellaneous

An Epidemiological Study To Evaluate the Incidence of Activated Protein C Resistance in the General Population Using a Polymerase Chain Reaction-Mediated Restriction Fragment Length Polymorphism Assay: Implications for the Critical Care Patient

G. J. Tsongalis, W. N. Rezuke, and A. H. B. Wu

Abstract

Thromboembolic episodes are responsible for a significant number of patients requiring critical care, affecting approximately 1 in 1000 subjects annually. Pulmonary embolism alone accounts for 50–100000 deaths per year in the United States, with more than 50% of these being elderly. Genetic resistance to activated protein C (APC) is the most common inherited disorder associated with a predisposition for thrombosis. A missense mutation has recently been identified in the gene coding for coagulation factor V (codon 506) which renders this procoagulant factor resistant to inactivation by APC, resulting in an increased risk for venous thrombosis. There is a five- to tenfold increased risk of thromboembolic disease in people who are heterozygous for this mutation, and a much greater risk for those who are homozygous. The prevalence of this mutation in patients with a history of thromboembolism is high (20%–50%), as is the prevalence in the general population (5%–10%). The ability to detect this mutation raises several questions concerning risk analysis. Are healthy individuals who have the mutation in the factor V gene predisposed to venous thromboembolism? Should prophylactic or more intense and prolonged anticoagulant treatment be administered to those who have the mutation? In an attempt to define the prevalence of this mutation in an in-house hospital patient population, we evaluated 397 randomly chosen patients for the factor V mutation using an established polymerase chain reaction (PCR)-mediated restriction fragment length polymorphism (RFLP) assay. Genomic DNA was extracted from whole blood and amplified using factor V exon 10-specific primers. Amplified factor V was digested with the *Mnl*I restriction endonuclease. The mutation destroys a restriction enzyme recognition site, resulting in altered restriction fragments which are detected by polyacrylamide gel electrophoresis. In our study, we found one patient homozygous and 16 patients heterozygous for the factor V gene mutation, which is an overall incidence of 4%. These results are comparable to those reported by others. We have demonstrated that this PCR-mediated RFLP assay is a simple and reliable method of evaluating patients for the presence of resistance to APC. Further prospective studies are needed to evaluate the clinical significance of this genetic alteration in otherwise asymptomatic patients.

Introduction

Venous thrombosis is a major medical problem worldwide, with an annual incidence of approximately 1 in 1000 individuals; it represents a major cause of morbidity and mortality [1]. Mortality most commonly results from associated pulmonary embolism, for which epigenetic risk factors have been identified, including the precipitating factors of major surgery, trauma, oral contraceptive intake, pregnancy, prolonged immobility, and obesity [1]. Genetic risk factors have also been identified which result in thrombophilia, the familial tendency to develop thromboembolic disease. These risk factors include inherited deficiencies of protein C, protein S, and antithrombin III, which are physiologic inhibitors of blood coagulation [1–8]. Together, these deficiencies account for only 5%–15% of thrombophilia cases. Thus, until recently, the etiology of 85%–95% of familial cases has been indeterminate.

In 1993, Dahlback et al. [9] described a defect in the protein C-related coagulation pathway as an inherited resistance to the anticoagulant action of APC, which is now known to account for the majority of cases of inherited thrombophilia [9]. Protein C is a circulating anticoagulant and is a very important regulator of hemostasis [1]. Protein C circulates in plasma as an inactive zymogen and is converted to APC by thrombin. APC mediates its anticoagulant effect by inactivating factors Va and VIIIa, which are cofactors involved in the intrinsic and extrinsic coagulation pathways (Fig. 1). Inherited resistance to APC occurs in most cases because of a single point mutation in the gene for factor V, which results in a simple amino acid substitution in the factor V protein (Fig. 2) [10]. The altered factor V protein resists inactivation by APC and results in an increased risk for thrombosis. In contrast to hereditary deficiencies of protein C, protein S, and antithrombin III, which are relatively uncommon, inherited resistance to APC is quite common. Studies have suggested that APC resistance may be up to ten times more common than any of the other known hereditary deficiencies. In patients with a history of thrombosis, APC resistance may occur in as many as 50%–60% of cases [1–3, 10, 11].

The objective of this study was to determine the prevalence of this mutation in a randomly chosen patient population without knowledge of prior history and in a series of patients with a clinical history of hypercoagulability using a PCR/RFLP-based assay. We also demonstrated that this mutation can be detected by heteroduplex analysis of PCR-amplified products as a complimentary screening method. In addition, we present three clinical profiles of patients who were genotyped for the factor V mutation at the request of their physician.

Materials and Methods

Specimens

Peripheral blood samples from 397 randomly chosen patients, collected in lavender ethylenediaminetetraacetic acid (EDTA) vacutainer tubes for prior

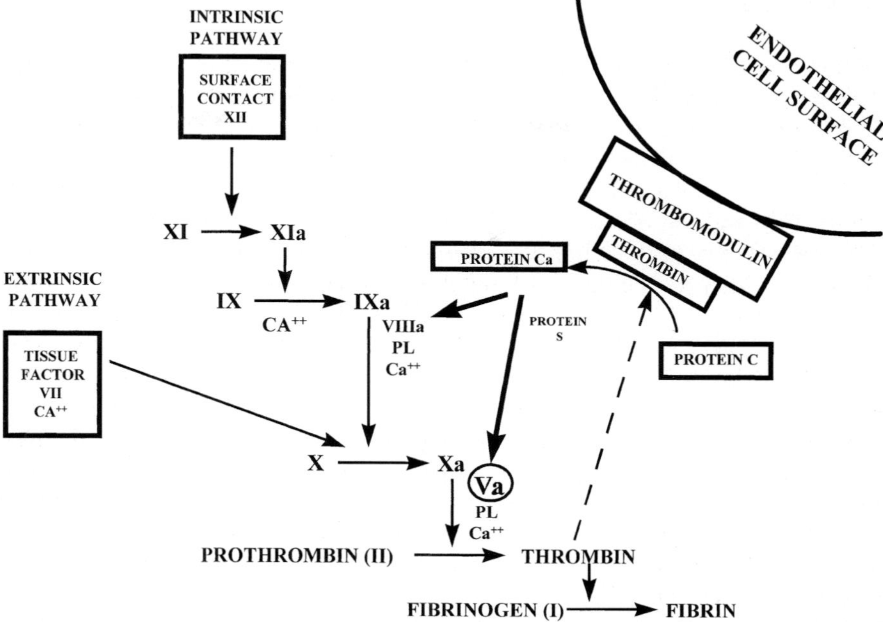

Fig. 1. Extrinsic and intrinsic coagulation pathways, highlighting pathways of inactivation by activated protein C. *PL*, phospholipid

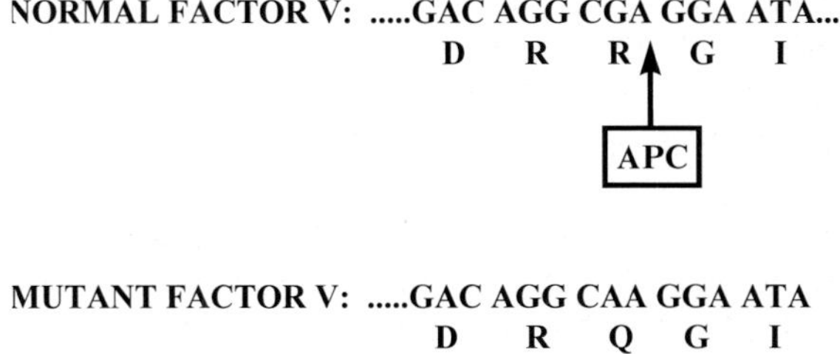

Fig. 2. Normal and mutant factor V gene sequences with corresponding amino acid sequences. The activated protein C (*APC*) cleavage site is indicated in the normal sequence, but is not present in the mutant due to a single point mutation which results in a change of amino acids

complete blood cell (CBC) evaluation, were obtained from the Hematology Laboratory for analysis of the factor V mutation. All samples were stripped of patient identifiers before being processed. In addition, 95 blood samples were obtained from individuals with a history of hypercoagulability for mutation analysis. Cases reported here as selected case studies were chosen from those submitted to the Molecular Pathology Laboratory for clinical evaluation of the factor V mutation. Medical histories on these patients were received from the attending physicians.

DNA Extraction

DNA was extracted from peripheral blood leukocytes using a nonorganic, high salt extraction protocol. Whole blood cells were initially lysed in hypotonic lysis buffer (0.64 M sucrose, 0.02 M Tris-HCl, pH 7.6; 0.01 M $MgCl_2$, 2% Triton X-100). A nuclear pellet was retrieved by centrifugation and resuspended in 3 ml nuclear lysis buffer (10 mM Tris-HCl, pH 7.6; 400 mM NaCl; 2 mM EDTA; 0.5% sodium dodecyl sulfate, SDS) prior to digestion with 290 µg proteinase K/ml at 37°C for 3 h. DNA was then ethanol precipitated after the addition of saturated NaCl and resuspended in 10 mM Tris, 1 mM EDTA (pH 7.6).

Polymerase Chain Reaction

Genomic DNA (0.5–1.0 µg), isolated as described above, was incubated in a total reaction volume of 50 µl containing 150 ng of both the forward and reverse exon specific primers, 2.5 units Taq polymerase, 200 µM each deoxynucleotide triphosphate, 1.5 mM $MgCl_2$, 10 mM Tris-HCl (pH 8.3), 50 mM KCl, and 0.001% gelatin. The primers used were as follows: 1691G forward primer, 5′-ACC CAC AGA AAA TGA TGC CCA-3′ and 1691G reverse primer, 5′-TGC CCC ATT ATT TAG CCA GGA-3′ [11]. DNA was initially denatured at 94°C for 5 min prior to amplification in the Perkin Elmer 2400 or 9600 thermocyclers. PCR amplification was accomplished using 35 cycles consisting of 30 s of denaturation at 94°C, 30 s of annealing at 55°C, and 30 s of extension at 72°C. The final cycle included a 7-min extension step at 72°C.

Restriction Endonuclease Digestion

The mutation associated with APC resistance destroys an *Mnl*I restriction enzyme recognition sequence and is thus detected by digestion of PCR-amplified products with this enzyme (Fig. 3) [11]. The restriction digestion was performed in a total volume of 50 µl and consisted of 30 µl PCR product, 14 µl dH_2O, 10 units *Mnl*I enzyme (New England Biolabs, Beverly, MA), and 5 µl 10X buffer. Samples were then incubated for 3 h at 37°C. Restriction fragment size analysis was performed by visualization of digested PCR products after separation by gel electrophoresis in a 10% polyacrylamide gel and staining with ethidium bromide.

Heteroduplex Screening Assay

An aliquot of PCR-amplified product from each patient was combined with PCR-amplified product from a known normal control sample and heat-denatured at 100°C in a beaker of water for 5 min. Samples were then slowly cooled to 45°C by allowing the sample to remain in the water at room tem-

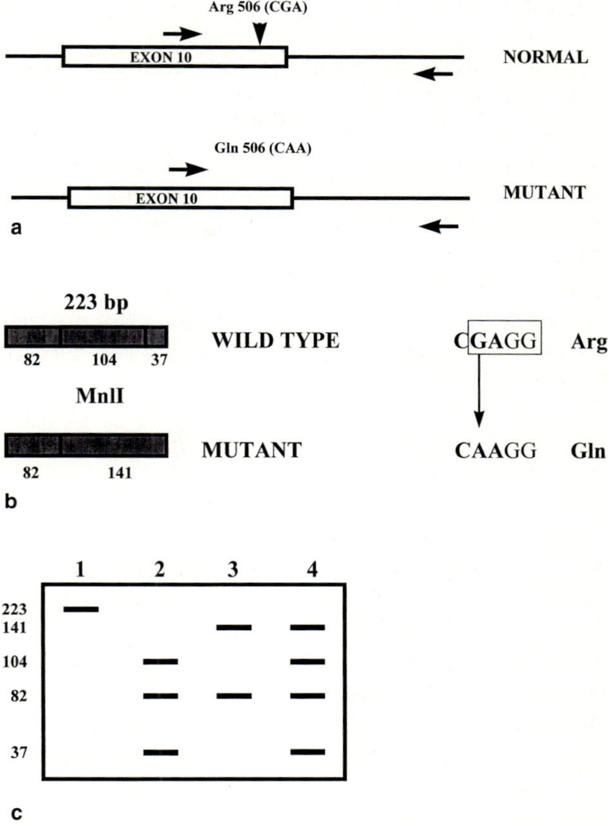

Fig. 3. a Direct detection of the G to A point mutation in exon 10 of the factor V gene is performed by a polymerase chain reaction (PCR)-mediated restriction fragment length polymorphism (RFLP) assay. Primers (*arrows*) which flank the region of the mutation (*arrowhead*) are used to amplify a 223-bp fragment which is subsequently digested with the *Mnl*I restriction endonuclease. **b** *Mnl*I restriction digestion map of the 223-bp fragment associated with activated protein C resistance. Fragment sizes for normal (wild-type) and mutant sequences are given below the 223-bp amplified product (in bp). Normal and mutated sequences are shown (*right*). The *Mnl*I recognition sequence (*box*) is altered by the mutation, as is the amino acid codon sequence (*boldface*). **c** The mutation is subsequently detected by gel electrophoresis, as the mutation destroys a digestion site for this enzyme. *Lane 1*, undigested PCR product; *lane 2*, normal individual; *lane 3*, homozygous mutant; *lane 4*, heterozygous mutant

perature on the benchtop. An aliquot of 40 µl of this product was mixed with 6 µl gel loading buffer and electrophoresed on a 38-cm vertical Hydrolink-MDE gel (FMC, Rockland, ME). The MDE gel was diluted to a 1X concentration in 0.6X Tris-borate + EDTA (TBE) and 15% urea. Subsequent to gel polymerization, electrophoresis was carried out for 16 h at 500 V. The gel was stained with ethidium bromide in TBE and then photographed under ultraviolet light.

Results

We determined the prevalence of the factor V mutation in our institution's patient population by examining 397 randomly chosen blood samples. Each sample was obtained after all clinical laboratory tests had been completed, and each was stripped of all patient identifiers to maintain confidentiality and randomness. DNA was extracted and APC resistance determined by a PCR-mediated RFLP assay which identifies the factor V mutation (Fig. 3). This mutation results from a single base change, G to A transition, which replaces Arg with Gln at amino acid residue 506. This alteration also results in the destruction of an *Mnl*I restriction endonuclease recognition site, which makes this mutation easy to detect by direct molecular analysis and gel electrophoresis (Figs. 3, 4).

In this assay, a homozygous normal or wild-type allele consists of a banding pattern which includes 104-bp, 82-bp, and 37-bp fragments. A homozygous mutant will consist of a banding pattern which includes only 141-bp and 82-bp fragments due to the loss of an *Mnl*I restriction enzyme recognition site. A heterozygous pattern is recognized as having 141-bp, 104-bp, 82-bp, and 37-bp fragments (Figs. 3, 4). We were able to identify 16 heterozygotes and one homozygote in 397 randomly chosen patient blood samples for an overall incidence of approximately 4% (Table 1). Of 95 patients who had a previous history of a thrombosis-related event, 23 (24%) were heterozygous for this mutation (Table 1). We were also able to demonstrate that detection of heteroduplex formation of PCR-amplified products was suitable for identifying the presence of this mutation without restriction enzyme digestion (Fig. 5). This may be used as a complimentary screening procedure for detection of the factor V mutation.

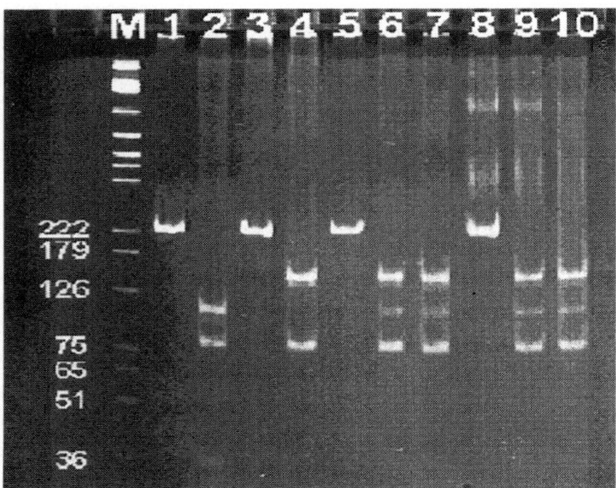

Fig. 4. Polyacrylamide gel electrophoresis of undigested (*lanes 1, 3, 5, 8*) and digested (*lanes 2, 4, 6, 7, 9, 10*) polymerase chain reaction (PCR)-amplified exon 10 of the factor V gene. *Lane M*, molecular size marker (sizes given in bp on the *left*). *Lane 2*, normal; *lane 4*, homozygous mutant; *lanes 6, 7, 9, 10*, heterozygous mutants

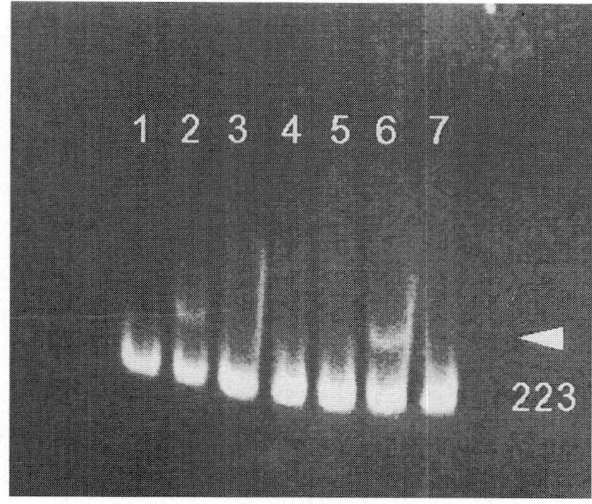

Fig. 5. Heteroduplex analysis for the factor V Leiden gene mutation. *Lanes 1, 3–5, 7,* normal 223-bp fragment; *lanes 2, 6,* heterozygous heteroduplex pattern. *Arrowhead* indicates heteroduplex fragment which migrates slower than normal fragment

Table 1. Prevalence of the factor V gene mutation in random patients and patients with a clinical history (HX) at Hartford Hospital

Group	Patients (n)	Heterozygotes	
		(n)	(%)
Random	397	16	4.0
Clinical HX	95	23	24

Of the initial 15 specimens received in our laboratory for evaluation for APC resistance as part of an evaluation for hereditary thrombophilia, four (27%) were heterozygous for the factor V gene mutation (Table 2) and included three females and one male. Clinical histories were obtained from three of these patients. The first case was a 69-year-old man who presented with an acute myocardial infarction secondary to a coronary artery thrombosis. This patient also had a prior history of deep venous thrombosis. The second case involved a previously healthy 58-year-old postmenopausal woman who was participating in an estrogen replacement therapy study. Within 2–3 weeks of being placed on exogenous estrogens, she developed a pulmonary embolism. The third case was that of a 43-year-old woman who had a prior history of a hysterectomy and who subsequently developed a pulmonary embolism while on oral contraceptives. She also had a past history of thrombophlebitis and a family (father) history of death due to pulmonary embolism.

Table 2. Patient demographics of a population of patients at risk for developing thrombosis and results of the factor V gene mutation analysis

Case no.	Age	Sex	Mutation analysis
1	63	F	Normal
2	58	F	Heterozygous
3	56	F	Normal
4	46	F	Normal
5	43	F	Heterozygous
6	42	F	Heterozygous
7	40	F	Normal
8	33	F	Normal
9	76	M	Normal
10	74	M	Normal
11	69	M	Heterozygous
12	58	M	Normal
13	53	M	Normal
14	43	M	Normal
15	15	M	Normal

Discussion

The pathophysiology of thrombosis was first described in the nineteenth century by Virchow, who hypothesized that a combination of alterations in blood flow hemodynamics (stasis), injury to the blood vessel wall, and abnormalities in blood coagulability were the three critical ingredients leading to clot formation [12]. The cascade of events which results in formation of a fibrin clot can be classified into two major pathways, the intrinsic and extrinsic pathways, which are summarized in Fig. 1 [1]. Both pathways are downregulated by the action of protein C. The protein C anticoagulation system is initiated by the binding of thrombin to thrombomodulin, an endothelial surface membrane protein. Thrombin then cleaves circulating protein C, resulting in the activation of protein C to form APC. APC exerts its anticoagulant effect by inactivating activated factor V (Va) and activated factor VIII (VIIIa). Protein S and phospholipid serve as cofactors to APC in this reaction. Loss of factor Va cofactor activity results from cleavage at Arg-506 by APC, and complete inactivation of factor Va is thought to require an additional cleavage at Arg-306. In contrast, a single cleavage by APC at Arg-562 of factor VIIIa results in complete inactivation. Factors Va and VIIIa increase the catalytic activity of factor Xa and thus thrombin formation by more than 1000-fold. Therefore, it is easily recognized that resistance to inactivation by APC would result in increased hypercoagulability.

In 1993, Dahlback et al. [9] analyzed patient plasmas from a group of patients with a history of thromboembolic disease. By performing a modified partial thromboplastin time assay through the addition of APC, a group of patients with a lowered anticoagulant response to APC were identified [9, 13]. In 1994, Dahlback and Hildebrand [14] attributed this resistance to APC to the reduced cofactor activity of factor V. Bertina et al. [10] later demonstrated that resistance to APC was attributable to a single point mutation in the factor V gene. This G to A missense mutation, commonly referred to as factor V Leiden or Arg-506 Gln, substitutes arginine with glutamine at amino acid residue 506 and renders factor Va resistant to cleavage by APC (Fig. 2). The vast majority of thrombophilia patients with resistance to APC have been identified as having this factor V gene mutation, which is inherited as an autosomal dominant trait [13]. Individuals who are heterozygous for this condition have a five- to tenfold increased risk of venous thrombosis, while those who are homozygous have a 50- to 100-fold increased risk [15].

Hereditary resistance to APC is now considered to be the most common cause of thrombosis, a common clinical dilemma for which there is now a direct molecular assay. The PCR-mediated detection of a single G to A point mutation is easily achieved, because the point mutation results in loss of a known *MnlI* restriction site. We have demonstrated that, in addition to the established PCR-mediated assay, the factor V gene mutation can be detected by assaying for heteroduplex formation. The molecular assays offer several advantages over the traditional functional assays available for APC resistance. Functional or clot-based assays for APC resistance are difficult for laboratories to establish, because there is a need for extremely careful standardization. These assays require testing of many normal control specimens to establish a normal range, and reported results from heterozygotes and normal individuals often overlap. More importantly, this assay cannot be performed on patients who are receiving anticoagulant therapy or in patients who may have an elevated partial thromboplastin time (PTT) for a variety of other reasons. The functional assays are less costly and thus seem better suited for screening protocols. The molecular assay is now, however, considered the gold standard for detecting APC resistance due to its extremely high sensitivity and specificity.

The laboratory detection of APC resistance is very significant for the critical care patient considering the high prevalence of this disorder and the potential for prevention of thrombosis with anticoagulant therapy. We have described random screening of hospitalized patients in whom the heterozygous mutation was detected in approximately 4% of patients tested. Only one of 397 patients was homozygous for this mutation. The increased prevalence of this mutation in an asymptomatic population suggests that other factors may be involved in the development of thrombosis. In heterozygous patients, thrombotic episodes may occur when other associated genetic, physical, or biochemical risks are present in addition to the factor V gene mutation. The simultaneous occurrence of two independent risk factors has given rise to a "two-hit" hypothesis for coagulation. This is in some ways similar to the two-hit hypothesis commonly associated with inactivation of tumor suppressor genes [16], which also applies to the factor V gene. Acquisition of a mutation in the second factor V allele increases the risk of developing thrombosis five- to tenfold for a heterozygote and 50- to 100-fold for a homozygote. It is well established that associated deficiencies of protein C, protein S, and antithrombin III also increase the risk for thrombosis. Samaha et al. [2] demonstrated that, in a cohort of pregnant women, 28% developed a thromboembolic event who were also resistant to APC, compared to 44% for antithrombin III, 24% for protein C, and 16% for protein S deficiencies. Heterozygotes who experience major trauma (i.e., accidental, surgical) or who take certain types of medications may also be at increased risk.

The majority of cases of APC resistance described thus far have been associated with the development of venous thrombosis. Whether the factor V gene mutation increases an individual's risk for arterial thrombosis has not been well established. Ridker et al. [11] evaluated approximately 15000 healthy men for this mutation to determine the risk of developing arterial thrombosis associated with myocardial infarction or stroke. In this study, the presence of the factor V gene mutation was not associated with the development of arterial thrombosis, but was associated with complicating venous thrombosis. It is still not clear whether this mutation predisposes an individual to arterial thrombosis when other risk factors are also present. In one of our cases, the patient was found to be heterozygous for the factor V gene mutation and presented with myocardial infarction secondary to coronary artery thrombosis. Whether these events are related is unclear and certainly warrants further studies.

It is now recognized that primary venous thrombosis has a genetic component and that the most common alteration, a mutation in the factor V gene, is easily identifiable. It is conceivable that patients who are found to have the factor V gene mutation be placed on prophylactic anticoagulant therapy. Therapies may either be short-term or long-term and include oral anticoagulants such as heparin or warfarin (Fig. 6). Dahlback suggests that treatment of patients with the heterozygous mutation and without a personal or family history of thromboembolic disease should consist in prophylactic anticoagulant therapy only in clinical situations associated with provoking thrombosis [1]. Patients with recurrent thrombosis are treated more aggressively for an extended period. During the fiscal year 1995 at our institution, 66 patients and 45 patients had a principle diagnosis of pulmonary embolism and deep venous thrombosis, respectively. The average length of stay per patient was 7.6 days for pulmonary embolism patients and 6.1 days for deep venous thrombosis patients, with average charges to the patient of approximately $ 10000 and $ 8200, respectively. If 25% of patients with a prior history of thromboembolic episodes have the factor V gene mutation and are treated prophylactically, this could mean cost savings of more than $ 250000 for the health care system and a decrease in length of stay by approximately 200 days. Although these figures represent crude outcome data, it is obvious that more detailed outcomes studies are warranted for a disease-causing mutation of such high prevalence.

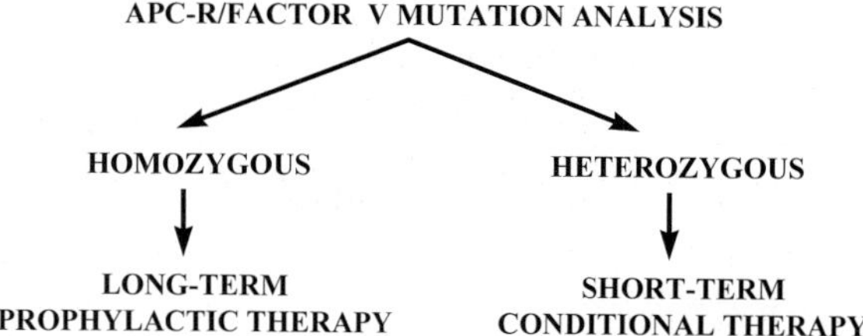

Fig. 6. Clinical management of the factor V mutant, activated proteint C-resistant (*APC-R*) patient

The full spectrum of clinical manifestations associated with this factor V gene mutation is still unknown in the asymptomatic population: Are healthy individuals who have the mutation in the factor V gene predisposed to venous thromboembolism? Should prophylactic or more intense and prolonged anticoagulant treatment be administered to those who have the mutation? Is the mutation associated with other pathophysiologic events? Unlike many other genetic alterations, the biochemistry of the factor V gene mutation is well understood and the results treatable. However, the consequences of a factor V gene mutation in the general population without history of thrombosis must be further evaluated.

References

1. Dahlback B (1995) Inherited thrombophilia: resistance to activated protein C as a pathogenic factor of venous thromboembolism. Blood 85:607–614
2. Samaha M, Trossaert M, Conrad J, Horellou MH, Elalamy I, Samama MM (1995) Prevalence and patient profile in activated protein C resistance. Am J Clin Pathol 104:450–454
3. Liu XY, Nelson D, Crant C, Morthland V, Goodnight SH, Press RD (1995) Molecular detection of a common mutation in coagulation factor V causing thrombosis via hereditary resistance to activated protein C. Diagn Mol Pathol 4:191–197
4. Griffin JH, Evatt B, Wideman C, Fernandez JA (1993) Anticoagulant protein C pathway defective in majority of thrombophilic patients. Blood 82:1989–1993
5. Dahlback B (1994) Physiological anticoagulation: resistance to activated protein C and venous thromboembolism. J Clin Invest 94:923–927
6. Comp PC, Nixon RR, Cooper MR, Esmon CT (1984) Familial protein S deficiency is associated with recurrent thrombosis. J Clin Invest 74:2082–2088
7. Bauer KA (1994) Hypercoagulability: a new cofactor in the protein C anticoagulant pathway. N Engl J Med 330:566–567
8. Demers C, Ginsberg JS, Hirsh J (1992) Thrombosis in antithrombin III deficient persons: report of a large kindred and literature review. Ann Intern Med 116:754–761
9. Dahlback B, Carlsson M, Svensson PJ (1993) Familial thrombophilia due to a previously unrecognized mechanism characterized by poor anticoagulant response to activated protein C: prediction of a cofactor to activated protein C. Proc Natl Acad Sci USA 90:1004–1008
10. Bertina RM, Koeleman BP, Koster T et al (1994) Mutation in blood coagulation factor V associated with resistance to activated protein C. Nature 369:64–67

11. Ridker PM, Hennekens CH, Lindpaintner K et al (1995) Mutation in the gene coding for coagulation factor V and the risk of myocardial infarction, stroke, and venous thrombosis in apparently healthy men. N Engl J Med 332:912–917
12. Virchow R (1856) Phlogose und Thrombose in Gefäßsystem. In: Virchow R (ed) Gesammelte Abhandlungen zur Wissenschaftsbereichen Medizin. Von Meideinger, Frankfurt, pp 458–636
13. Svennson PJ, Dahlback B (1994) Resistance to activated protein C as a basis of venous thrombosis. N Engl J Med 330:517–522
14. Dahlback B, Hildebrand B (1994) Inherited resistance to activated protein C is corrected by anticoagulant cofactor activity found to be property of factor V. Proc Natl Acad Sci USA 91:1396–1400
15. Zoller B, Svensson PJ, He X, Dahlback B (1994) Identification of the same factor V gene mutation in 47 out of 50 thrombosis-prone families with inherited resistance to activated protein C. J Clin Invest 94:2521–2524
16. Knudson AG (1971) Mutation and cancer: a statistical study of retinoblastoma. Proc Natl Acad Sci USA 68:820–823

Use of Thrombin Inhibitors Ex Vivo Allows Critical Care Clinical Chemistry and Haematology Testing on the Same Specimens

A. W. Lyon, S. R. Harding, D. Drobot, and M. E. Lyon

Introduction

The aim of this study was to evaluate the stability of the thrombin inhibitors D-phenylalanyl-L-prolyl-L-arginine chloromethylketone (PPACK) or argatroban for anticoagulation of blood prior to critical care testing of whole blood or plasma.

Methods

Initially we evaluated the effect of PPACK (0–200 µM) or argatroban (0–590 µM) on serum glucose, urea, creatinine, calcium and electrolyte tests on two chemistry analysers (Hitachi 717 and Ektachem 700XR). Subsequently, plasma and serum from whole blood samples containing either 15000 IU heparin/l or 75 µM PPACK or 245 µM argatroban or no anticoagulant were tested and compared. We analysed and compared whole blood containing either 75 µM PPACK or 245 µM argatroban or ethylene diamine tetra-acetic acid (EDTA) using a Coulter STK-R haematology analyser at intervals for 90 min.

Results

The measurement of electrolytes, urea, calcium or glucose was unaffected by either argatroban or PPACK in either serum or anticoagulant-specific plasmas ($p>0.05$). For specimens from individual donors, serum potassium was higher than plasma potassium, irrespective of the anticoagulant used. Clinically equivalent complete blood counts were achieved for 60 min using EDTA-whole blood or whole blood containing 245 µM argatroban or 75 µM PPACK. However, automated differential white cell counting was not reliable with either form of thrombin inhibitor-whole blood. Argatroban-anticoagulated blood demonstrated concentration- and time-dependent changes in platelet counts, whereas platelet counts were stable in blood containing 75 µM PPACK for up to 90 min.

Conclusions

Specimens of blood anticoagulated with either 75 µM PPACK or 245 µM argatroban can be used for either critical care chemistry or haematology testing.

A Clinical Case of Transitory Diabetes Mellitus During Lyell Syndrome

C. Sandrine, B. H. Limam, K. Limam, Y. Braham, S. Bouchoucha,
and A. Miled

Introduction

Lyell syndrome or toxic epidermal necrosis is a severe reaction of the skin characterised by a widespread erythema and detachment of epidermis resembling scalding. It carries a high mortality rate and is most often provoked by a wide variety of drugs. Systemic signs of the disease include high fever, leucocytosis, elevation of transaminases, albuminuria and water and electrolyte imbalance, which may proceed to haemodynamic shock, pulmonary oedema and renal failure. We describe a case of Lyell syndrome which was accompanied by diabetes mellitus.

Methods

The patient was a 28-year-old woman who developed Lyell syndrome after taking a number of drug medications, including lincomycin, niflumic acid and lysin acetyl salicylate. She presented with a major portion (45%) of her skin detached and she was admitted to the intensive care unit.

Results

The initial electrolyte, renal function and glucose results were all within the reference range. On day 2, the plasma glucose had increased to 12.3 mmol/l, and by day 4 it was 20 mmol/l. At this time the patient also had a metabolic acidosis (HCO_3, 18 mmol/l) with an anion gap (26 mmol/l) but normal lactate (1.8 mmol/l). The patient developed a polyvisceral cytolysis with abnormal enzyme activities, which were maximal on day 3 and were as follows: aspartate aminotransferase (AST), 229 IU/l; alanine aminotransferase (ALT), 121 IU/l; creatine kinase (CK), 17940 IU/l; CK muscle-brain (CK-MB), 10 IU/l; amylase, 44 IU/l. At the same time, the patient was noted to have a leucopaenia (2900/µl) and thrombocytopaenia (50000/µl), which was thought to be due to the drug medication.

The patient did not improve until day 9, when there was progressive improvement with normalisation of the plasma glucose and amylase by day 13 and spontaneous regression of the rhabdomyolysis. By day 25, all biochemical parameters were within the reference range, and the patient was discharged on day 30.

Conclusions

This case of Lyell syndrome was unusual in that it was accompanied by diabetes mellitus and pancreatitis.

Parenteral Nutrition in Pre-Term Infants: Influence on the Development of Nephrocalcinosis

B. Hoppe, O. Datwyler, C. Holm, I. Forster, S. Fanconi, N. Blau, and E. Leumann

Introduction

Previous studies have shown that there is a higher risk of developing nephrocalcinosis in pre-term infants receiving parenteral nutrition (TPN) than in those receiving breastmilk nutrition. It was concluded from these studies that the nephrocalcinosis might be due to the amino acid solution in TPN. The aim of this study was to measure the effects on a number of urine parameters in babies given amino acid solutions.

Methods

A breastmilk-adapted amino acid solution (Vaminolact 6%) was given to eight pre-term infants of less than 1500 g birth weight and less than 35 weeks gestation (group 1). These infants were compared with 11 pre-term infants examined in a previous study who received an amino acid solution containing electrolytes (Vamin-Glucose 7%, group 2). On day 2 (period A) and day 3 (period B) and once between days 4 and 10 (period C), 24-h urine was collected for measurement of calcium, creatinine, oxalate and citrate. Urinary calcium/oxalate saturation was calculated by the computer programme EQUIL 2. Renal ultrasonography was performed every second week until discharge.

Results

Table 1 shows the calcium to creatinine, calcium to oxalate, calcium to citrate and oxalate to creatinine ratios during the different time periods in the two groups. The calcium to creatinine ratio increased significantly in group 1 ($p<0.05$), but remained lower than in group 2. The oxalate to creatinine ratio in group 1 was always higher than in group 2 ($p<0.05$). The calcium to citrate ratio increased significantly in group 1 ($p<0.05$), whereas only a slight increase was found in group 2. Calcium/oxalate saturation increased in both groups, but was higher in group 1 than in group 2 during period C ($p<0.02$).

Table 1. Urine parameters on day 2 (period A), day 3 (period B) and once between days 4 and 10 (period C) in pre-term infants given a breastmilk-adapted amino acid solution (group 1) and in pre-term infants given an amino acid solution containing electrolytes (group 2)

	Group 1			Group 2		
	Period A	Period B	Period C	Period A	Period B	Period C
Calcium/creatinine (mol/mol)	0.29		1.09*	0.62		1.35
Oxalate/creatinine (mmol/mol)	327	342	292	167*	167*	175
Calcium/citrate (mol/mol)	1.2		7.8*	1.8		3.45
Calcium/oxalate (mol/mmol)			4.61**			2.96

*$p<0.05$; **$p<0.02$.

The mean daily calcium, sodium and protein intake were comparable in the two groups, except for a lower protein intake in period A and a lower sodium intake in period C in group 1. There was a significantly higher phosphorus intake in group 2 ($p<0.05$). Nephrocalcinosis was later diagnosed ultrasonographically in two infants in group 1 and in one infant in group 2.

Conclusions

The breastmilk-adapted amino acid solution did not reduce the risk of nephrocalcinosis in pre-term infants on parenteral nutrition.

Arterial to Intramucosal pH Gradient Does Not Predict Mortality in the Intensive Care Unit

C.D. Gomersall, G.M. Joynt, T.A. Buckley, K.M. Ho, R.J. Young, and T.E. Oh

Introduction

Splanchnic ischaemia is postulated to be of major importance in the development of multi-organ failure and hence death in critically ill patients [1]. Low gastric intramucosal pH (pHi), which is thought to reflect splanchnic ischaemia, is associated with poor outcome [2]. However, low pHi may simply be a reflection of systemic acidosis [3] and the arterial pH (pHa) to pHi gradient may be a more specific indicator of adequacy of splanchnic oxygen delivery. The aim of this study was to examine the relationship between pHa-pHi gradient and mortality in the intensive care unit.

Methods

The study was carried out on 61 patients who were emergency admissions. Patients with brain injury, active gastrointestinal bleeding or aged less than 18 years and those in whom insertion of a nasogastric tube was contraindicated were excluded. Measurements of pHi, intramucosal PCO_2 ($PiCO_2$) and pHa were made at 0, 12 and 24 h using a gastric tonometer (Trip NGS, Tonometrics Inc., Hopkinton, MA) and a blood gas analyser (Ciba Corning 288). All patients were entered into this study within 6 h of admission to the intensive care unit, all received ranitidine (50 mg every 8 h) and none were enterally fed during the study period. Statistical analysis was performed using Student's *t* test, and *p* values were corrected for multiple significance using the Bonferroni method.

Results

The mean Acute Physiology and Chronic Health Evaluation (APACHE) score was 26, and the mortality rate in intensive care was 39%. Results for the various parameters measured in those who survived and those who died are shown in Table 1 together with the statistical significance.

Table 1. Gastric intramucosal pH (pHi), arterial pH (pHa), pHa-pHi gradient and intramucosal PCO_2 ($PiCO_2$) in survivors and non-survivors

	pHi			pHa			pHa-pHi			$PiCO_2$		
	0 h	12 h	24 h	0 h	12 h	24 h	0 h	12 h	24 h	0 h	12 h	24 h
Survivors	7.25	7.27	7.24	7.31	7.36	7.36	0.06	0.08	0.12	6.67	6.79	7.92
Non-survivors	7.12	7.27	7.20	7.20	7.30	7.30	0.08	0.03	0.10	8.05	6.91	8.58
p value	0.03	NS	NS	0.01	0.05	NS	NS	NS	NS	NS	NS	NS
Corrected *p* value	NS	NS	NS	<0.05	NS	NS	NS	NS	NS	NS	NS	NS

NS, not significant.

Conclusions

The pHa-pHi gradient has no prognostic significance, suggesting that either it does not reflect adequacy of oxygen delivery or that splanchnic ischaemia is not of major importance in determining mortality in the intensive care unit. The results also suggest, contrary to a recent report [4], that $PiCO_2$ is not a prognostic marker.

References

1. Fiddian-Green RG (1995) Gastric intramucosal pH, tissue oxygenation and acid-base balance. Br J Anaesth 74:591–606
2. Maynard N, Bihari D, Belae R et al (1993) Assessment of splanchnic oxygenation by gastric tonometry in patients with acute circulatory failure. JAMA 270:1203–1210
3. Boyd O, Mckay CJ, Lamb G et al (1993) Comparison of clinical information gained from routine blood-gas analysis and from gastric tonometry for intramucosal pH. Lancet 341:142–146
4. Friedman G, Berlot G, Kahn RJ et al (1995) Combined measurements of blood lactate concentrations and gastric intramucosal in patients with severe sepsis. Crit Care Med 23:1184–1193

Stapedial Reflex in Cephalic Tetanus

C. de Souza, D. R. Karnad, R. A. de Souza, A. Raje,
K. Mansukhani, and G. H. Tilve

Introduction

Tetanus is an acute and often fatal disease caused by an endotoxin produced by *Clostridium tetani*, and patients usually die due to exhaustion from generalised muscle spasms. Cephalic tetanus develops from injuries to the face with involvement of the cranial nerve. The stapedial reflex is the contraction of the stapedial muscle in response to auditory stimulus and is frequently used for impedance audiological evaluation. It has previously been used in the diagnosis of myasthenia gravis and Bell's palsy, and we report on the application of this reflex in three patients with cephalic tetanus.

Methods

In addition to the three patients with cephalic tetanus, we studied three patients with generalised tetanus and 50 normal controls. The stapedial reflex threshold (ipsilateral and contralateral ears tested at 500 Hz, 1 kHz, 2 kHz and 4 kHz) and the stapedial decay (ipsilateral and contralateral ears tested at 500 Hz and 1 kHz at intensity of 115 dB for 10 s) were evaluated. Clinical observation, pure tone audiometry and electromyography (EMG) were performed serially. The stapedial reflex was elicited with an impedance audiometer (Madsen impedance audiometer Z0174, New York) and was also done serially.

Results

The normal controls did not reveal stapedial muscle spasm. In patients suffering from generalised tetanus, stapedial spasms were seen but did not precede generalised spasms. EMG confirmed the presence of cephalic tetanus in our patients. All patients suffering from cephalic tetanus demonstrated stapedial muscle spasm. In cephalic tetanus, the facial muscles go through three phases, which were also demonstrated by the stapedial muscle but preceded the activity of the facial muscles. One patient had sustained stapedial muscle spasms and went on to develop severe generalised spasms, while the other two patients had ill-sustained spasms and developed less severe generalised spasms.

Conclusions

This study has demonstrated that spasms of the stapedial muscle do occur in tetanus and precede generalised muscle spasms by a few days. Furthermore, from the type of stapedial muscle spasm it was possible to predict the course of the disease and, more importantly, the onset of generalised muscle spasms. Thus we were able to take timely action to prevent deaths. This test was only done in three patients, but our observations suggest that this test has the potential to predict the onset and course of cephalic tetanus.

Springer
and the
environment

At Springer we firmly believe that an international science publisher has a special obligation to the environment, and our corporate policies consistently reflect this conviction.

We also expect our business partners – paper mills, printers, packaging manufacturers, etc. – to commit themselves to using materials and production processes that do not harm the environment. The paper in this book is made from low- or no-chlorine pulp and is acid free, in conformance with international standards for paper permanency.

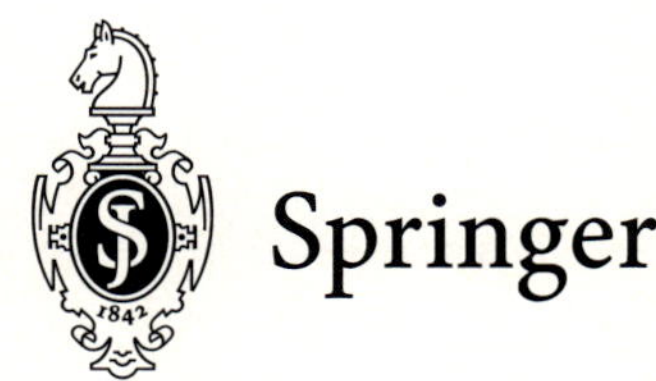

Springer

Printing: Saladruck, Berlin
Binding: Buchbinderei Lüderitz & Bauer, Berlin